John Arderon's *De judiciis urinarum*

EXETER MEDIEVAL TEXTS AND STUDIES

Series Editors: Vincent Gillespie and Richard Dance

Founded by M.J. Swanton and later co-edited by Marion Glasscoe

John Arderon's *De judiciis urinarum*

A Middle English Commentary on Giles of Corbeil's *Carmen de urinis*

in Glasgow University Library, MS Hunter 328 and Manchester University Library, MS Rylands Eng. 1310

Edited by

Javier Calle-Martín

LIVERPOOL UNIVERSITY PRESS

Contents

Illustrations

Possibly as a result of Payne's reply, or perhaps independently of it, Brockbank also wrote to George Warner about the Medical Society's manuscript. (He may actually have mailed it to each of his experts *seriatim*; the letters suggest they had looked at it directly.) In his reply of 16 January 1905 Warner did not have as much to say about the content of the manuscript as Payne had, but he did suggest that there were parallels in books 2 and 3 of an anonymous Middle English uroscopy in Sloane 2196. A week later, on 23 January, Warner sent Brockbank another note, saying "I doubt whether the Ms. treatise on urines which you [Brockbank] sent to me is worth publication". This note has the feel of something that Brockbank had asked about but that Warner had forgotten to mention in the first letter, rather than a gratuitous dig at the manuscript. It is a not entirely surprising judgement from the editor of facsimile editions of the Queen Mary Psalter, the Sforza Book of Hours, the Benedictional of Aethelwold, catalogues of the Royal and King's Collections, and other fine specimens of medieval book production.

One can imagine that Warner's second letter was a rather discouraging missive to receive, though Brockbank did at least prepare a public lecture on the manuscript, perhaps for his colleagues in the Medical Society: an outline and draft speaker's notes for that lecture are included in the envelope that now accompanies MS Eng. 1310. He may even have had lantern-slides made of some of the folios, judging from the speaker's notes, although those slides do not appear to have been preserved.

However, if Brockbank had looked north as well as south in his search for opinions about the manuscript – in particular, if he had sent a similar query to P. H. Aitken in Glasgow, who was in the process of completing John Young's catalogue of the Hunterian Collection (which appeared in 1908) – he might have received a very different answer about the identity and date of the text contained therein. Aitken would surely have recognised the text, as it also occurs, with additional Latin material but otherwise in a very close copy, even down to illustrations, on folios 1–44 of the fifteenth-century manuscript Hunter 328. The extra Latin passages include a first-person authorial prologue that gives the author's name and title, Master Johannes Arderon or Arderoun, physician of Henry IV; in the text proper, we find the appropriate lines of Giles de Corbeil's Latin *Carmen de urinis* for each of the 20 colours and 18 contents of urine treated by the main Middle English text, lines that are omitted in the Manchester volume. Aitken might then have mentioned the Manchester manuscript in the Hunterian catalogue, and the information could have become part of scholarly knowledge for the last hundred-plus years. It might even have resulted in Brockbank's undertaking of an edition of the text, potentially a worthy medical comrade to D'Arcy Power's more or less contemporary (1910; 1922) editions of surgical writings by Arderon's fourteenth-century near-namesake John of Arderne.

Now, however, Professor Calle-Martín has completed a much fuller edition than Brockbank would probably have attempted, giving us both the earlier Hunterian text and its Mancunian descendant (the two texts are so close, aside from sixteenth-century modernisations and abridgements in the later manuscript, that they must have some genetic relationship). This is a most welcome addition to the growing literature on Middle English medical texts, a field still very much in need of the editions on which future criticism and scholarship will be founded.

A few words about the importance of the work itself, titled by its author *De judiciis urinarum per colores & contenta*, are in order before moving on to the edition proper. Arderon's treatise on Giles's *Carmen de urinis* is one of the very rare instances of Middle English medical writing that takes the form of an academic commentary, with a primary text set out in a display script (in Hunter 328; as noted above, the Latin verses are omitted in Rylands 1310), surrounded by explanatory text in a smaller cursive script.[1] As such, the commentary is one of the most important examples of the transfer of learned medicine into Middle English and quite early among similarly learned works. Unlike most Middle English medical writers, Arderon clothes his treatise in traditional academic garb: a passage-by-passage commentary on a canonical text with extensive citations of authorities dating back to Hippocrates, including such medical luminaries as Galen, Theophilus, Isaac Israeli, Giles himself, Gilbertus Anglicus, Walter Agilon, Jean de St Amand and Bernard de Gordon.[2] To be sure, the Middle English text in Hunter 328 is only very generally keyed to the passages from Giles, in that each Latin passage treats a particular colour or content in urine, followed in Middle English by additional information about the colour or the content from a wide range of authorities. This is not the kind of commentary that gives short lemmas from the main text and then expounds them (as can be found in the unfinished *Commentary on the Hippocratic Prognostics* in Cambridge, Trinity College MS R.14.52, a translation from an as-yet-unidentified Latin original). But the visual rhetoric of a block of display text followed or surrounded by subordinate text in smaller script, so characteristic of commentaries in

[1] On the rarity of Middle English medical texts that take the form of a commentary, see Taavitsainen and Pahta 2001 and Taavitsainen 2004, though neither of these articles mentions the Arderon text.

[2] Arderon's list of authorities is remarkably similar to those cited in the uroscopic first treatise of the *Trifolium* written by Simon Bredon, Fellow of Merton College (c. 1310–1372), which survives only in Oxford, Bodleian Library, MS Digby 160, ff. 102r–222v (*tractatus* 1, ff. 103v–172v), though the Bredon text is not presented as a commentary on Giles's poem. Preliminary comparison of Arderon's text and the *Trifolium* shows that the Middle English treatise is not a direct translation of the Latin one, but does share at least some signs with it. For bio-bibliographic information on Bredon see Snedegar 1999, where the *Trifolium* is dated to the mid-1340s (290).

medieval manuscripts, is clearly behind the layout we find in Hunter 328. It may be that the omission of the Latin passages from Giles by the Rylands scribe reflects a recognition that the Latin verses were not actually necessary to understand the Middle English and that the Middle English does not directly explain Giles's sometimes cryptic Latin. Or it may simply be that the person for whom the Rylands version was made had no Latin, so *all* Latin material, including the prologue, was omitted. The Hunterian scribe and his implied audience must have valued the Latin more highly.

Another exceptional feature of this text is its amazing density of source citation throughout, much thicker than in any other Middle English uroscopic text I know, including such 'high academic' Middle English uroscopies as Henry Daniel's *Liber Uricrisiarum*, the several Middle English versions of Walter Agilon's treatise on the colours and contents of urines, the chapters on urine and uroscopy in Bartholomeus Anglicus and the uroscopic passages in the *Commentary on the Hippocratic Prognostics*. Whether the citations are all accurate or traceable to their alleged sources, however, is a question that must await future study, as must questions about possible intermediate source texts such as the *Liber Uricrisiarum*,[3] the Latin commentary on Giles by Gilbertus Anglicus, and English adaptations of uroscopies based on Walter Agilon.

Two other points about the commentary are worth making, in the hope that readers of this edition will find them suggestive for additional future research on the vernacularisation of medical knowledge in later medieval England. First, the relatively early date of the *De judiciis urinarum* and its inclusion of two less academic but more widely disseminated English uroscopies, the *Twenty Jordans* Series and components from the *Dome of Uryne*, must mean that those texts were already in circulation, in whole or in part, early in the fifteenth century. This is not a surprising conclusion, given the large number of fifteenth-century manuscripts of each work, but reassuring to find confirmed by Arderon's text. Second, the *De judiciis urinarum* offers additional evidence for an apparent flurry of Latin-sourced uroscopic translation and compilation in late fourteenth- and early fifteenth-century England. Instances include:

[3] Sampling Arderon's and Daniel's chapters on Black and Glaucus urines shows that relations between the two authors' works are complex. While there is relatively little parallel material in the two Glaucus chapters, much of Arderon's language in his chapter on Black urine (and even the order of his signs) bears striking verbal resemblance to the corresponding material in *Liber Uricrisiarum* book 2, followed by selected black urines from the "Rules of Isaac" chapter at the end of some copies of Daniel's work. Yet Arderon never mentions Daniel by name, and attributes many of the signs to the various Latin, Greek and Arabic authorities named in Simon Bredon's *Trifolium*, authorities not linked to the signs by Daniel. Further work is clearly needed to work out the intertextual relationships involved.

- Henry Daniel's *Liber Uricrisiarum* (c. 1377–1382);
- one of the translations of Walter Agilon's colours and contents treatise, preceded in one manuscript (CUL Ii.6.17) by a prologue attributing the translation to a Master Bartholomew, O.F.M., at the request of King Richard and Queen Anne (i.e. between Anne's coronation in 1382 and her death in 1394);
- the Seventeen-Chapter Abbreviation of the *Liber Uricrisiarum*, which was incorporated into the medical compendium compiled for Thomas Plawdon, probably the barber-surgeon of London who died before 1413;
- and the text that I have titled *Rufus Subrufus*, a 20-colour uroscopy preceded in four copies by a prologue that attributes its translation from Latin to "the wisest clerks in physic of England", said to be working at the behest of either Henry IV or Henry V, depending on the manuscript.

But investigation of relative datings of Middle English uroscopies and of a possible fashion for vernacular versions of learned urine texts in the late fourteenth and early fifteenth centuries, like deeper study of the sources that Arderon claims for his comments on Giles, can wait until scholars have had a chance to digest Professor Calle-Martín's parallel-text edition. The edition gives us complete access to both surviving copies of this important text, supported by thorough analyses of the linguistic, paleographic and punctuational features of those copies. These formal features will be of special interest to scholars and students of English historical linguistics, and Calle-Martín's extensive discussion provides valuable detail for future studies of the evolving orthography and punctuation of the late medieval to early modern period – significantly, spanning the opening decades of the print revolution.

In addition to dialect and paleographic analysis, Professor Calle-Martín provides readers with a glossarial treasure-house of medical terminology, from technical uroscopic vocabulary (often not included in the standard dictionaries) to names of illnesses, therapeutic materials and physiological processes, which will be of value to lexicographers and historians of medieval vernacular medicine alike. The occasional updatings of vocabulary in the Rylands copy of the text may also contribute to our understanding of early modern semantic change, particularly in a controlled field of discourse.

Most valuable of all, however, is simply having Arderon's text in print and available to modern researchers, in fields from English literature and language to the history of medicine and of the dissemination of Latinate learning into the vernacular. For those seeking a general introduction to the leading diagnostic method of medieval and early modern medicine, Arderon's "judgements of urines by colours and contents" offers both the

pulsibus and Theophilus' *De urinis*, to which Corbeil himself added some material from Isaac Judaeus (more commonly referred to as Isaac Israeli nowadays).[2]

Corbeil's *Carmen de urinis* served as the base text for *De judiciis urinarum*, a late ME commented version of Corbeil's original. The witness begins with a statement referring to Master John Arderon, the physician of King Henry IV, as the main authority of the book. Despite the similar names, there does not seem to be any likely identification of John Arderon with the reputed physician John of Arderne, as suggested in some early references to the question of authorship.[3] Different arguments have been proposed to reject Arderne's authorship. On the one hand, there is an obvious chronological mismatch, as "the reference to the physician of King Henry IV, who was already dead, shows that it must have been written after the year 1413, and Arderne was born in 1307" (Power 1913: 129). On the other, the impersonal style and high degree of academic content of the Hunterian witness differ from Arderne's other attributed writings (Tavormina 2014: 99).

The date of composition of the treatise definitely helps to shed some light on its authorship. According to Tavormina, "if Arderon had been *medicus domini regis* to Henry IV, then it seems likely that the writing took place sometime in the early 15th century (ante-1425)" (2007a). Thus, the reference to John of Arderne must have been taken either as a copyist's error or as a reference to some other John of Arderne living in the fifteenth century. Getz proposes a John Arderne the Younger, probably a member of the same family, who was accused of having murdered John Crophill of Annesley, but unfortunately no further details of his trade or profession are currently known (1990: 263; also Tavormina 2014: 99–100). There are other Ardernes in the historical records of the period, but again it is not possible to ascertain a definite authorship, as this surname was an extremely common one in the fourteenth century, "and there is no good reason for connecting him to any of the other John Ardernes found in contemporary documents" (Jones 2004; *Oxford Dictionary of National Biography*, s.v. *John Arderne*).

[2] Tavormina highlights the use of verse "as a mnemonic aid for practical instruction [...] in both the Latin and the vernacular realms of medieval learning" and, in view of this fact, "Giles of Corbeil's verse treatise on urines was an equivalent of a medical best-seller from its appearance in the early thirteenth century onwards" (Tavormina 2010: 592).

[3] Even though Power disregards this possibility in his introduction to his edition of the *Fistula in ano*, there is still room for ambiguity. While on pages xii and xiii he acknowledges that "there is nothing to show that [Arderne] was living in the reign of Henry IV" and that the Commentary was "clearly written after 20 March, 1413", he eventually seems to attribute the Commentary to Arderne again on page xv (Power 1910). Some years later, however, Power clearly stated that "Arderne could have never been the author of the Commentary, although the name of Arderon might well be a copyist's error" (1913: 129).

1.2. The English version of *De judiciis urinarum*

In line with Corbeil's original text, the English version of *De judiciis urinarum* is a detailed uroscopic treatise instructing the mediaeval practitioner on the examination of urine with 20 colours and 18 to 19 contents (Tavormina 2007b: 647). It incorporates colour descriptions, diagnoses, medicines and information about urinary contents. The author, however, does not confine himself to mere commentary, as he also incorporates material from two well-known uroscopic traditions. On the one hand, the text is accompanied by drawings of urine flasks with captions providing the ailments associated with a particular colour together with recommended medicines needed for treatment. These flask diagrams have been taken from *The Twenty Jordan* series, a text widely circulated in the period and preserved in more than 60 manuscripts (Tavormina 2005: 45–49). On the other hand, the text concludes with two modified components of the *Dome of Urine*, another uroscopic compendium preserved in more than 50 manuscripts (Calle-Martín 2013: 243–274). From the 17 parts of the *Dome of Urine*, the author selects two and appends them at the end of the treatise.[4] Plates 1 and 2 reproduce the very first folios of this version, illustrating the Latin introduction together with some of Giles's Latin and Middle English, and a pair of flasks.

In addition to these two popular ME uroscopies, the English version includes extensive citations of medical authorities in the field of uroscopy, such as Hippocrates, Ptolemy, Galen, Isidore of Seville, Theophilus, Israeli, Avicenna, Averroes, Giles of Corbeil, Gilbertus Anglicus, Walter Agilon, Bernard de Gordon and Jean de Saint Amand, which corroborate the medical lore and level of expertise of the ME commentator. Arderne's reference to the authorities and the use of the conventions of academic discursive models becomes more than an obsession in the sense that "the name-dropping of academic authorities is thicker here than in any other Middle English uroscopic text" (Tavormina 2007a).

The English vernacular tradition of *De judiciis urinarum* has been preserved in two different witnesses (Tavormina 2014: 100). The first – Glasgow, Glasgow University Library, MS Hunter 328, ff. 1r–44v (henceforth *Hu*), early fifteenth century (Cross 2004: 26) – includes the Latin text of Giles of Corbeil's *Carmen de urinis*, accompanied by the commentator's reformulation in the vernacular. Both commentaries and compilations, according to Taavitsainen, are genres at the learned end of the scale of science with an important difference between them. While in compilations opinions are attributed to others without taking sides, commentaries cross-refer to other texts in such a way that conflicting views

[4] The author appended the four sentences on substance and several signs of death from "Urine Troubly with Clouds" (Tavormina 2014: 100).

are presented in order to reconcile them, the commentator's voice being then heard in the conclusions (2004: 40–44; 2005: 185). Essentially a Latin genre, commentaries did not proliferate much in ME medical and academic discourse, and the few examples available show that they did not strictly follow the Latin conventions of the genre.[5] The text in *Hu* is not constrained by the content of the Latin original in terms of the colour or the content of the urine. Quite the contrary: the commentator provides additional pieces of information referring back to a wider set of authorities and, more importantly, preserving his authorial voice and, at the same time, controlling the readers' perception of the text. Formally speaking, this version complies with the rhetoric of other commentaries in mediaeval manuscripts, where the Latin and the vernacular texts are clearly distinguished by a different script (Tavormina 2007a).

Apart from Arderne's commentary on Corbeil's *Carmen de urinis*, the Hunter copy also houses two other treatises of unknown authorship: *An Alphabetical List of Remedies* (ff. 45r–62r) and *An Alphabetical List of Medicines* (62v–68v), written in the same hand throughout. The recipes contained in this witness include lists of plants, herbs and other substances for the preparation of plasters, medicines, salves, syrups and so on (Sánchez-Reed 2010).

The second witness – Manchester, Rylands Library, MS Rylands 1310, ff. 1r–21r (henceforth *Ry*), early sixteenth century (Ker 1983: 427) – leaves out the Latin material, housing an eModE version of Corbeil's *De judiciis urinarum*. Even though the formal requirements safely comply with those of a sixteenth-century English text, particularly on phono-orthographic grounds, this copy is closely connected to the Hunterian witness in terms of content.

Unlike the previous version, *Ry* omits the embedded quotations of Giles's Latin text together with some of the marginal structural indicators. The omission of the Latin material is open to different interpretations. The copyist could have decided to omit it in view of the following facts: a) that Latin was unnecessary to follow the vernacular version of the text; b) that there is no direct connection between the Latin verses and the ME rendering; and c) that the copyist did not have a full command of Latin (Tavormina 2007a; Tavormina 2014: 100). Whatever the motivation might have been, *Ry* concentrates on the vernacular material, therefore omitting the authorial statement at the beginning, together with Giles's Latin verses, and incorporating the line drawings of urine flasks found in the Hunterian witness, as shown in Plate 3.

[5] Vernacular uroscopies, however, traditionally follow the commentary tradition; both Walter Agilon's *Commentarium urinarum* and Henry Daniel's *Liber uricrisiarum* can be safely ascribed to this tradition (Taavitsainen 2004: 52–55).

In spite of the close resemblances between the two witnesses,[6] it is difficult to postulate that *Ry* is a lineal (or a collateral) descendant of *Hu*. This is also Tavormina's argument in the foreword to the present edition, where she affirms that "the two texts are so close, aside from sixteenth-century modernisations in the later manuscript, that they must have some genetic relationship". In this vein, it is safer to propose the existence of a common ancestor to both copies, possibly fairly close to *Hu* in terms of both date of composition and content, which later descends in two separate, though closely parallel, lines to *Hu* and *Ry*, this being the origin of their genetic relationship (Tavormina, personal communication).

The early Modern English scribe takes the role of a translator who transfers the contents of the source text into fluent and understandable sixteenth-century English (Pahta and Taavitsainen 2004: 13). This objective leads him to the use of frequent omissions and alterations for the sake of a better understanding of the statement. Example (1a–b) reproduces the beginning of blue urine, where the early Modern English copyist voluntarily discards the reference to *adustioun* and *mortification*, assuming that it is sufficiently explained in the following statement. The copyist in example (2a–b), in turn, alters the position of *souch* to modify the noun *urin* suggesting the existence of an error in the source text.

> (1a) Bloo colo*ur*. or ledy. or wan colo*ur*. all in on. lyke toward white. *and* black. havyng oneþys more of þe black þan of þe white. somtyme it betokenyth. adustyon. and somtyme Mortifycacion. Whan it aperyth w*ith* a grenesse it betoken*yth* adustyon / and if þ*er* apere noo*n* it betokenyt Mortifycacion. *secundu*m theophilu*m*. & Egidiu*m*. (*Hu*, f. 3v)

> (1b) Bloo color or ledy or wan colour al is on like towarde white and blac having onethis more of the blac than of the white a grenesse it betokneth adustio*un*. And if ther appere non it betoknyth mortification *secundu*m theophilu*m* and Egidiu*m*. (*Ry*, f. 2v)

> (2a) þ*er*ffor all*e* such maner*e* of /froth\ vryn betokenyth eu*er* ventosyte. towh. *and* viscouse humeris. i*n* þe body. ysaac. (*Hu*, f. 31r)

> (2b) therfor al man*er* of souch frothy vrin tokneth euer ventosite touh and viscouse humeres in the body Ysaac. (Ry, f. 15r)

[6] In an email to the Keeper of Manuscripts and Archives at the Rylands Library (dated 4 September 2006), Tavormina concludes that "the English texts are very close in the passages I was able to compare, from the beginning, middle and end".

Muhammad Ibn Zakariya al Rhazes (865–925), more commonly known by his Latin names Razus, Rasis or Rhazes, was a Persian alchemist, philosopher and physician reputed as a leading figure in the history of medicine. He combined the teaching of medicine with his activity as a chief physician in Baghdad. Rasus not only followed Hippocrates and Galen but also extended the analytical procedures of his predecessors. In the field of urology he was most interested in the "pathophysiology of the urinary tract, venereal diseases, and kidney and bladder calculi" (Ashtiyani and Cyrus 2010: 106). He is best known for his book *Al-Hawi*, a medical encyclopaedia subsequently translated into Latin as *Liber continens*, where he deals, among many other medical issues, with the anatomy and physiology of the urinary tract and kidneys and, more importantly, with how to diagnose the related diseases (Shamsi, Haghverdi and Ashtiyani 2014: 278).

Ibn Sina (c. 980–1037), latinised as Avicenna, is one of the most significant figures of the Islamic Golden Age. He was the author of more than 400 works, of which just 240 have been preserved; the list includes works of astronomy, earth sciences, mathematics, logic, physics, philosophy and medicine, among other subjects. Like other Arab medical writers, Avicenna continued the tradition of Greek scientific medicine, using uroscopy for prognostic and diagnostic purposes. His most significant contribution was *The Canon of Medicine*, which became one of the most important medical texts in many universities until the seventeenth century. Avicenna's system of urine inspection considered aspects such as colour, density, turbidity, sediment, quantity, froth and odour (Afnan 1958: 201–206).

Inb Rushd (1126–1198), in Latin Averroes, was a mediaeval Andalusian polymath who wrote on logic, philosophy, theology, astronomy, mathematics, physics and medicine, among other subjects. He wrote a medical encyclopaedia on general medicine that was translated into Latin with the name of *Colliget*, together with a compilation of the works of Galen and a commentary on Avicenna's *Canon of Medicine* (Fakhry 2001: 124–126).

Giles of Corbeil (c. 1140–1224), as mentioned above, wrote *Carmen de urinis*, the Latin original that served as the base text for *De judiciis urinarum* and the object of the present edition.

Gilbertus Anglicus (c. 1180–c. 1250), also known as Gilbert of England, was an English physician known especially for his *Compendium medicinae*, in which he drew together the basics of surgery and medicine at that time. It is considered to be among the major works of early mediaeval medicine, "representing the oldest complete treatise on general medicine written by an English author which has survived to the present day" (Esteban-Segura 2012: 17). The uroscopic content is conveniently dealt with in the sections concerned with the liver, the spleen, the kidneys and the bladder, towards the end of the *Compendium*.

Both Walter Agilon (c. 1250–1306) and Bernard de Gordon (1270–1330) practised medicine in Montpellier. Agilon was a master of medicine there and the author of "*Summa medicinalis*, in which uroscopy plays a central role, and a *Compendium urinarum*, in which he elaborated on the earlier writings on the subject" (Prioreschi 2001, IV: 579; also Diepgen 1911; O'Boyle 1998: 113–114). De Gordon was a French doctor and professor of medicine who studied in Salerno before his teaching activity in Montpellier. He is best known for his *Lilium medicine sive de morborum prope omnium curatione* ('The lily of medicine or the cure of almost all diseases'). Bernard de Gordon was also the author of *Libellus de impregnatione* ('Small book of pregnancy'), *Arbor ægritudinum* ('Book on diseases'), *Opusculum de authenticis urinarum signis* ('Small work on the authentic urinary symptoms'), and *De cautelis urinarum* ('Cautions concerning urine') (Prioreschi 2001, IV: 383–384).

Jean de Saint Amand (c. 1262–1312) was a thirteenth-century French physician who combined tradition and renewal. He wrote commentaries on the texts that formed part of the Parisian curriculum at that time, such as *Antidotarium Nicolai*, Hippocrates' *Prognostics and Regimen on Acute Diseases*, Isaac Israeli's *De dietis*, Philaretus' *De pulsibus* and Theophilus' *De urinis*, as well as introducing new texts, such as *Revocativum memorie*, *De flebotomia* and *De viribus plantarum* (Jacquart 1994: 195; Wickersheimer 1979: 476–477), mostly relying on the Galenic tradition.

Taking into account the number of authorities cited in *De judiciis urinarum*, it would be desirable to identify the specific sources for individual items attributed to the various authorities in order to ascertain the English medical writers'/translators' awareness of major medical authorities. Such source analysis, however, is not within the scope of the present edition, which is mostly concerned with the synoptic presentation of the hitherto unedited English vernacular versions of this uroscopic treatise, so that it may be used as the source text not only in Historical Linguistics but also in other areas, such as Textual Criticism, Codicology, Palaeography and the History of Medicine.

1.4. The language

The orthography of the period 1400–1660 is characterised by the establishment of a written standard throughout the country (Blake 1996: 12). This standard has been traditionally explained using the single ancestor dialect-hypothesis, which proposes a unitary source for Standard English based on the language of the East Midlands (Hope 2000: 49). In contrast with the single dialect-hypothesis, the appearance of Standard English is now widely interpreted as the confluence of various systems. Samuels proposes the 'Central Midland Standard' as the first literary standard, which was based on the spelling systems of Northamptonshire, Huntingdonshire and Bedfordshire (Samuels 1963; Blake 1996: 169).[7] This spelling system was later amalgamated with other alternative spellings emanating from the Chancery and from other influential bodies, such as the Privy Seal, Signet offices, law offices, ecclesiastical bodies and business centres, as well as from the contributions of individual writers who incorporated their own dialect forms into this emerging standard. As a result of these converging influences, a written standard emerged in the fifteenth century intended for wider use and the general public, which was thus deprived of conspicuous dialectal features (Nevalainen 2006: 29; McIntyre 2009: 21–22).[8] The uniformity, however, was observed to be greater in morphology than in orthography at this early stage.[9]

This standardisation is defined by the Milroys as an ongoing process of the suppression of optional variability in the quest for "functional efficiency of the language where misunderstanding should be reduced to the minimum, and efficiency enhanced to the maximum" (Milroy and Milroy 1999: 18–19; also Rutkowska 2013: 45). In itself, the formation of a vernacular standard is not a straightforward process, and different stages are identified in its implementation: selection, acceptance, diffusion, maintenance, elaboration of function, codification and prescription (Milroy and Milroy 1999: 22–24; Nevalainen and Tieken-Boon van Ostade 2006: 274–286).[10]

As far as scientific writing is concerned, this typology of writing progressively adapted to this new standard from the late fourteenth century with the adoption of what Taavitsainen calls the Central Midland spelling system in scientific texts (2000: 131). The process, however, differed from that observed in administrative and literary writing. The contribution of the Chancery Standard becomes less prominent in scientific writings from the late fifteenth century as a result of its implicit prestige, the learned status of this kind of prose making it less disposed towards the adoption of new spelling variants (Taavitsainen 2000: 146–147).

[7] The growing influence of this variety has been justified in sociohistorical terms in view of immigration to London and good transport and communication connections, eventually giving rise to the concentration of the Central Midland type in the capital (Blake 1996: 173).

[8] This Chancery form "assumed its mature form by 1430, and the written form spread throughout the country for official and business correspondence by the 1460s" (Poussa 1982: 81).

[9] On morphological grounds, this uniformity is initially attested in the use of the *-d* spelling for the past tense or the adoption of *th*-forms for third person plural pronominals, among others (Poussa 1982: 81).

[10] The role of these stages in the process of standardisation of English is discussed in detail in Nevalainen and Tieken-Boon van Ostade (2006: 274–286).

1.4.1. MS Hunter 328

The language of *Hu* is a typical case of the amalgamated Central Midland spelling system in the light of the evidence provided by the fit-technique in *A Linguistic Atlas of Late Mediaeval English* (henceforth *LALME*) (McIntosh et al. 1986; Benskin 1991: 9–26). The mapping of the orthographic variants allows the restriction of the geography of *Hu* towards the north of Northamptonshire, in the Central Midlands. Its linguistic profile (henceforth LP) is closely related to LP 737, a copy of the *Treatise on Seven Deadly Sins*, ascribed to this same origin (McIntosh et al. 1986, III: 369).[11]

The level of spelling standardisation, however, can be assessed by considering the weight of the variants that are not intrinsic to the Central Midland standard. In her analysis of the *Corpus of Early English Medical Writing* (1375–1550, c. 500,000 words), Taavitsainen proposes evaluating the orthography of the typical core features of the Central Midland Standard (2000: 137), which were initially proposed by Samuels (1963). The list includes variants such as *sich* 'such', *mych* 'much', *ony* 'any', *silf* 'self' and *stide* 'stead', to which we have added other features from LP 737 for accuracy. Of these, three core forms stand out (*such*, *much* and *any*) for not having a Central Midland form in Westminster usage. These forms are *sich*, *mich*, or *ony*, which "point to either an immigrant from Central Midlands, or a writer looking directly to the Central Midlands for his model" (Taavitsainen 2000: 137; also Benskin 1992: 92). For comparison, the abridged LPs of MSS Hunter 328 and Sussex College 55 are reproduced, where the variant forms of the Chancery Standard are given in bold:

- Glasgow University Library, MS Hunter 328: ***such ((suche))***, ***moch ((moche))***, *from*, *ech*, *ony*, *many*, *thouh*, *aȝens (ayens)*, *ȝytt*, *whan*, *throuh (through)*, *self*, *ȝeue (yeue)*, *without ((withoutyn))*, *togeder*, *nyȝh*.
- Cambridge, Sidney Sussex College, MS 55 (LP 737): ***suche (such)***, ***moche*** *(mekyl) moch*, *from*, *eche ((ech))*, *ony* ***((any))***, *many*, ***þough***, ***ageyn*** *(aȝens)*, *ȝit*, *whan (whanne)*, *þurgh*, *self*, ***geven***, *wiþ-oute ((wiþ-outen))*, *to-gidre*, *nyȝ*.

In strictly qualitative terms LP 737 presents a more advanced stage of standardisation, with the incorporation of more Chancery English lexemes. Notwithstanding the fact that the forms *such(e)* and *moch(e)* have already replaced the Central Midland forms *sich/swich* and *mich/mych* respectively in both witnesses, the Cambridge manuscript presents some recessive forms of the Central Midland standard, such as a) the Chancery English spelling *any*, which appears together with the constrained Central Midland form

[11] This treatise is found in Cambridge, Sidney Sussex College, MS 55 (Δ.3.10).

used in a contracted form denoting an omitted *e*, especially in those cases where the following word begins with a vowel or the consonant <h>, regardless of its pronunciation, whether silent or not, as in *thurin* > *the urin*, *thede* > *the hede*.

Inflectional morphology, on the other hand, also corroborates the incipient stage of the text in the standardisation continuum. Unlike spelling, traditionally viewed as displaying a greater variability, morphology is generally more susceptible to the influence of the standard. Trudgill mentions a set of morphological features that were soon adopted by the Chancery standard – among others, the third-person inflection in the present tense, the absence of present plural *-n* in verbs and the preference for *-ly* adverbs (1999: 125–126; Fisher 1996: 49–51). The analysis of these features may certainly shed some light on the level of regularisation of inflectional endings to the Chancery standard.

The third person singular inflection shows an outstanding preference for the inflections *-eth* (×347) and *-ith/-yth* (×90) in examples such as *diuideth*, *draweth* vs *smellith*, *stynkyth*, among others. These figures confirm the dominant role of the East Midland inflection in the Chancery Standard during this early stage of standardisation.[16] In addition, the scribe recurs to the inflections *-ø* (×54) and *-e* (×39) in instances such as *begin*, *put*, *stink* vs *blede*, *loke*, *pisse* and so on. Interestingly enough, the text does not show traces of the *-(e)s* inflection, considered in itself a typical diffusion of the latter half of the sixteenth century in the light of the evidence provided by the *Corpus of Early English Correspondence* (Nevalainen 2000: 349–252). As far as the substantive verb is concerned, the conjugation of the third person singular is clearly dominated by *is* (×462), while the variant form *be* (×134) is receding as a result of the general standardisation of the former.

The present indicative plural perfectly corresponds to the standard insofar as it is conjugated with the inflections *-ø* (×23), *-eth/-yth* (×6), *-e* (×5) and *-en* (×3), as in the cases of *cal*, *likneth*, *fastith*, *comyth*, *apere* and *sayn*, respectively. As shown, finite verbs in the plural have already lost part of their morphological richness as a consequence of the inflectional simplification that had already started in late ME. In the light of this, the Midland inflection *-en* is virtually obliterated in the text in favour of the other variants, the inflectionless form predominating in the conjugation of lexical verbs. The plural form of the verb *to be*, however, is still reluctant to adopt the northern form *ar* (×4), preferring the forms *be* (×45), *ben* (×14) and

16 The choice of these verbal inflections, however, seems to depend heavily on particular lexemes in the sense that some verbs are more prone to combine with *-eth* (e.g. *betokneth*) while others prefer the inflection *-ith/-yth* (e.g. *commyth*). The former stands out for being the most frequent lexical verb in the text, which perhaps distorts the degree of standardisation of this inflection in the sixteenth-century text, there being less difference between the two forms.

bene (×2), respectively. This actually complies with Nevalainen's findings in the *Corpus of Early English Correspondence*, where the traditional southern plural form *be* is the choice, while the generalisation of *are* did not take place in London until the latter half of the sixteenth century (2000: 348; Nevalainen and Tieken-Boon van Ostade 2006: 293).

Adverbs of manner are generally formed with the suffixes *-ly* (×64) and *-li* (×5), irrespective of the native or non-native origin of the lexeme, as in *sotelly, principally, fully, esyli, specialli, meneli* and so on. The *-e* and zero forms of the adverb are also witnessed in examples such as *abrode, sore* and *foul*, albeit with a sporadic occurrence. More important, however, is the absence of the adverbial suffix *-liche* in the text, a form that was soon deprived of standard recognition.

1.5. Codicology

1.5.1. Ownership

Like the other items in the Hunterian collection of manuscripts, *Hu* originally belonged to the personal library of William Hunter (1718–1783), an eighteenth-century reputed physician and surgeon who collected a number of books, manuscripts and artefacts, most of them scientific in nature (Porter 1985: 7–9). After his death in 1783 his library and other collections were bequeathed to the University of Glasgow, but they remained in London until 1807 for the use of his nephew Dr Matthew Baillie (1761–1823), also a physician.

According to the information published in the Rylands Library online catalogue, *Ry* was formerly owned by the Manchester Medical Society and later deposited with Owens College (later the University of Manchester) in 1875 under the supervision of Thomas Windsor, the librarian of the Manchester Medical Society from 1831 to 1910.

1.5.2. Material, dimensions and ink

Hu is written on a well-preserved vellum. The modern binding of the volume has protected it from damage over time, the only defects being some original vellum imperfections, as shown in f. 43r, which has a hole 26mm in diameter in its external margin. The volume is still characterised by a number of ink stains at the external bottom corners as a result of a continuous turning of the pages, the most conspicuous examples being found from f. 34r to 48v. In addition to this, the folios are, in general, "all gnawed off (by beetles) where not cropped" (Young and Aitken 1908: 264).

Even though originally displaying 69 folios, *Hu* has in its present form 68 folios, written in a single column of about 29 lines each. Written in an octavo size, the volume's dimensions are 196mm × 135mm, although there is some variation between folios.[17] Black ink is systematically employed for the running text. The writing is retouched in some places, as shown at the beginning of the volume, where the copyist refers back to the main authority of the text, Magister Iohannes Arderon (f. 1r). Red is used as a macro-textual device to highlight an important piece of information within the running text. The copyist makes use of vermilion in the following situations: a) to introduce the title and opening lines of a new section/subsection; b) to signal, with a rubricated initial, the beginning of a major section (some just touched with vermilion); c) to refer back, with red underlining, to the authorities of the text; d) to draw the *paragraphus*, the symbol employed to mark off the beginning of a new subsection in the text; and e) to highlight some of the marginal annotations.

Ry contains a total of 22 folios of well-preserved paper measuring 305mm × 215mm. The volume is not bound and for that reason the corners of some folios are damaged and cropped by the passing of time, f. 6r being an illustrative example. Like the Hunterian witness, this copy is rendered in black and red ink. The former is systematically used for the running text while the latter is exclusively used in the following contexts: a) section titles; b) rubricated initials indicating the beginning of a section;[18] c) the *paragraphus*, the symbol employed to mark off the beginning of a new subsection in the text; d) obliterations, longer ones in particular; and e) pagination, reproduced at the top right corner.

1.5.3. Quiring and collation

According to my personal inspection of the Hunter copy, the folios of the manuscript are distributed in nine quires with the following characteristics (Young and Aitken 1908: 264):

> Three paper fly-leaves (i^{3}). || I^{8}–3^{8}, $4^{7(8)}$, 5^{8}–7^{8}, $8^{7(8)}$, 9^{6}. || Three paper fly-leaves (ii^{3}). 4, 6. is cut out (probably to remove a miswritten leaf, as the text is continuous); 8, 3 is a half sheet (probably so originally).

Foliation is modern, written in pencil at the top right corner of the folios. The scribe makes use of catchwords, whereby the first word of a quire was written at the bottom of the last leaf of the preceding quire (Petti 1977: 6). *Hu* presents the characteristic octavo folding wherein quires consist of eight leaves each (Johnston 1945: 68), with the exception of irregular quires. Catchwords are not systematic in the volume, some of them being absent

17 Its dimensions are in accordance with the standard proportions of that particular type of folding in the period (Johnston 1945: 69).

18 Depending on their importance, these rubricated initials may take two, three or five lines.

as a result of the cutting of the folios before binding. The catchwords are in f. 8v (*glaukk*), f. 16v (*ruffe*), f. 24v (*under stonde*), f. 39v (*ward*) and f. 47v (*water of Rose*).

Ry, on the other hand, displays 21 folios distributed in three different quires, the last one containing just five folios. According to the collation of the Rylands Library, it was originally composed of 22 folios; the last one is now lacking, although this fact does not affect the reading of the manuscript as it was probably blank (I–2^8, $3^{5(1)}$). In addition to foliation, written by the scribe in red ink at the top-right corner, the folios of each quire are numbered in the lower right margin of the page in black ink to secure the correct sequencing of the material before binding. Thus, they are arranged using the first letter of the alphabet followed, in turn, by a Roman numeral in such a way that the first folios of the treatise are ordered with the following notation: *ai*, *aii*, *aiii*, etc.

1.5.4. Fly-leaves

Ry shows no fly-leaves at either the beginning or the end. According to the collation provided by Young and Aitken (1908: 264), *Hu* has two paper fly-leaves at the beginning (i^2) and two at the end (ii^2). On rebinding in 1958, however, a third paper fly-leaf was incorporated at the beginning and at the end, which explains my collation as i^3 and ii^3, respectively.

In i^3v, Dr Hunter's own handwriting makes reference to the scientific authority of the treatise, the prestigious practitioner John Arderon. The bottom part of this same fly-leaf records an old shelfmark of the volume in the Hunterian collection (2.7.16 bis), together with the one now in use (U.7.22, written in blue pencil).

> Magistri Iohannis Arderow | Opusculum de judiciis urinarum | per colores et contenta (a) | A collection of Recepts or Cures | for various disorders. English. | in the inscription is dñi regis illustris | principis Henricis quarti, so that we may presume this writer lived about the year 1400.

1.5.5. Ruling

Hu presents traces of frame-ruling drawn with brown crayon. The writing surface, however, varies consistently across the folios from 133mm (f.43r) to 141mm (f. 19r). The width of the folios is more consistent (86mm). The witness, however, does not show the use of line-ruling, a frequent device in other mediaeval prose compositions to ensure that the text has a visually appealing layout. As a result of this, the scribe is not consistent with regard to the number of lines per folio, which range from 24 (f. 31v) to 30 (f. 8v).

The Textualis component consists of a pre-defined set of letters common to the vast majority of manuscripts written in this style, leaving small room for the scribe to reshape the inventory (Roberts 2005: 161–164). The following letters characterise the Anglicana script: the two-compartment <a> (1); the loopless <d> (4); the single-compartment <g>, with occasional horns (7); the 8-shaped <s>, exclusively word-finally (20); and the two versions of letter <r>, the short and right-shouldered one (17) and the 2-shaped alternative (18), the latter exclusively after vowel <o> and other letters with a bow (see Derolez 2003: 138). The cursive component, in turn, predominates in the text as a result of the larger contribution of the Anglicana Formata. The most distinctive cursive letterforms are the following: the loop at the right side of the letter <b> (2); the absence of infralinear <f> (6); the (occasional) hooked ascender of the letters <h> (8) and <l> (11); the three-stroke <m> (12) – a feature that sharply differentiates the Anglicana Formata from the single stroke Anglicana (Derolez 2003: 138); long <s> in initial and medial positions (19); the long-approach stroke of the letter <v> (24) together with the conventional form of the letter <x> (26). The grading of the Secretary script, on the other hand, is witnessed in the use of two letters. First, the scribe discards the looped and three-shaped final stroke <w> of the Anglicana in favour of the simpler version of the Secretary, thus resembling a double <v> (25). Second, the text adopts the use of the three-stroke <e> (5) instead of the conventional Anglicana two-stroke form (Derolez 2003: 137).

In addition to the scribal hand, this version incorporates some marginal and superscript annotations together with textual corrections, Latinate pieces in particular. They are rendered with a legible early sixteenth-century script characterised by a commonplace Elizabethan Secretary hand, plausibly from the second half of that century on account of the use of particular letterforms, such as the v-like <r> or the long hooked form of <s>. The letter <c>, for instance, presents the characteristic horizontal stroke at the top of the crescent with the absence of the foot serif and the letter <g> is reproduced with the head as a semioval and the infralinear loop converted into a simple tail.

Ry is written with a commonplace sixteenth-century Elizabethan Secretary hand on account of the use of particular letterforms, which help the palaeographer to establish the early sixteenth century as a probable date of composition with some level of accuracy (Lester 1985: 66). Fig. 2 reproduces the full inventory of letters in *Ry*, where several items have been singled out for descriptive purposes.

The letter <a> shows the conventional shapes of Elizabethan penmen, both with the oval body open at the top (2) and with an oblique supralinear

both f. 1r (*The Latin verses in the Book are those of Egidius de Urinis (W3) [a monogram for? W.B.]*) and f. 44v (*The end of the Treatise of Urines*).

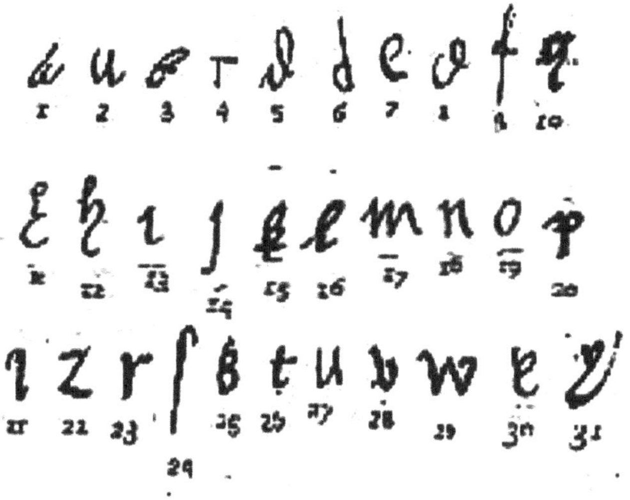

Fig. 2. Inventory of letterforms in *Ry* (adapted from Petti 1977: 17)

descending stroke (1), the latter a recurrent scribal practice by the end of the century (Petti 1977: 17). The letter <c> is rendered with a short vertical stroke together with a thin horizontal stroke at the top (4). The letter <e> is written with the open reversed vowel (8) as well as with its regular form (7), the latter perhaps as a relic of the fifteenth-century hybrid scripts. There are not, however, any contextual reasons governing the use of one or the other. Following the secretary alphabet, the letter <g> shows a semioval head with an infralinear upward loop (1). The shape of the letter <h> is variously represented by Elizabethan penmen, the variants differing "in the gradual reduction of the looped stem to a mere bow, in the elimination of the second semioval, and in the acquisition of a sinuous infralinear tail" (Tannenbaum 1930: 47), as in (11) and (12). Denholm-Young describes a characteristic gradient of this letter for the purposes of identification in the sense that "in the first half of the period the letter *h* is still half above the line. As time wears on it sinks lower and lower" to such an extent that three-quarters of the letter is below the line in the later Secretary hands (1954: 71). In this particular case, the letter does not extend much beyond the line of writing, which speaks for the early sixteenth-century composition of the treatise. The letter <r> also presents two versions, the 2-shaped (22) and the left-shouldered form (23), even though the former is significantly more frequent, irrespective of its position within the word. The letter <s> also presents two renderings: the long-hooked form (24) and the beta-like <s> (25); the former in initial and medial position, whereas the latter is preferred word-finally (see also Calle-Martín 2011: 46–48).

1.6.2. Marginalia

Marginalia is used for different purposes in the witnesses. Apart from the inclusion of longer insertions, the main function of the external margins in *Hu* is macro-structural, serving as a kind of index so that the reader can easily identify the key topics of the treatise. The list includes information ranging from chapter numbers to uroscopic terms, particular diseases and remedies, as shown in *de alba et aquosa vrina* (f. 7v), *þe dropesy* (f. 6r), *medicina* (f. 5r) and the like. Fig. 3 reproduces this macro-textual function, where these annotations have been rendered with the same hand as the running text:

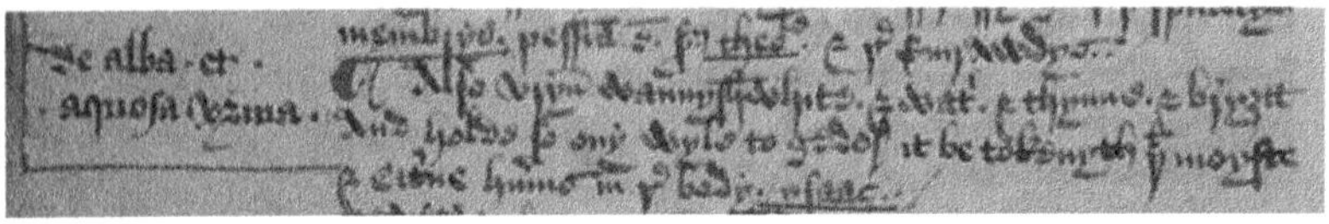

Fig. 3. Marginalia in *Hu* (f. 7v)

Following its mediaeval source, the marginal annotations in *Ry* also have macro-textual functions, although they are more sporadic. The early modern scribe sometimes ignores some of the information contained in the source text, being more committed to the inclusion of uroscopic terms and chapter numbers. This explains the constrained role of these marginal annotations in the early modern version (Fig. 4).

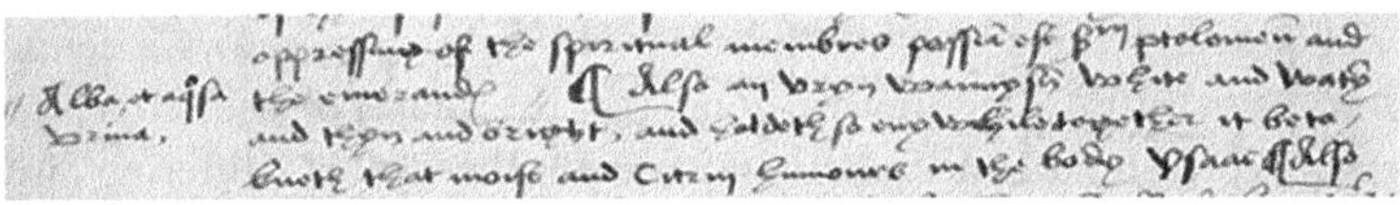

Fig. 4. Marginalia in *Ry* (f. 4v)

1.6.3. Punctuation

The repertory of punctuation marks differs in both witnesses. *Hu*, as a late ME composition, displays a rather constrained system, with the use of just two marks of punctuation. *Ry*, on the other hand, presents a more complex system with an inventory of seven symbols, which is the result of the increasing specialisation of punctuation in eModE documents, both written and printed. In both versions, however, there is a consistent scribal practice responding to a flexible and premeditated set of rules, mostly conceived to render grammatical relationships. Thus, the preference for the structural dimension of punctuation in both witnesses is surely associated with the particularities of this text type as academic compositions originally written to be read silently, hence the importance of grammatical relations.[21] This section reports on the uses and functions of marks of punctuation in both witnesses, distinguishing the different relationships of punctuation marks, whether macro-textual, sentential, clausal or phrasal.[22]

1.6.3.1. MS Hunter 328

Hu does not present a complex system of punctuation, especially if compared with other late ME scientific compositions (Alonso-Almeida 2002: 207–232; Calle-Martín 2004: 407–422; Calle-Martín and Miranda-Garcías 2005a: 27–44). The text is rendered with just two punctuation marks: the paraph mark (¶) and the punctus (.).

- *The paraph mark*: the paraph performs a macro-textual function by introducing the commentaries taken from the different authorities, which are often rendered one after the other in paragraph format. With a total of 534 instances in the text, this symbol then serves as a visual device, making it easier for the reader to find a particular diagnosis and its cure in the text. Example (3) shows the paraph heading the statements by Avicenna, Isaac and Hippocrates in the description of black urine:

> (3) ¶ and it it be thyke and inequal it betokenyt roryng. and hurlyng. and dystemperyng in þe body. euermore in such party as þu seyst it in þe vryn so is it in þe body. auicenna. 4º. ¶ Vryn blak weþer it be equal. or inequal if it be with a lytel body þat is lytel in quantyte. significat mortem. ysaac. ¶ also an vryn þat is moche. and derke. and dymme. swart betokenyt mortifycacion þan it is more blakker þan whan it is of þe waryssyng of þe feuer quarteyn. ypocras. (f. 2r)

The paraph is also used to introduce an important piece of information for the understanding of the topic. In example (4), the scribe recurs to this symbol to introduce the definitions of the terms *mortification*, *adustion* and *melancholy* as the causes of black urine:

> (4) [...] blak vryn is causyd of. iij thyngys. i. because of adustion. 2. because of mortificacion. 3. or with niger humour. id est. Malencoly.

[21] A new ideal of punctuation originates in the period, as it "ceases to be regarded primarily as a guide to the spoken language and becomes an aid to clarity in the printed work" (Salmon 1999: 40).

[22] It should be noted, however, that historical punctuation is not always consistent from beginning to end, as there are often counterexamples that may erroneously lead to the conclusion that punctuation is haphazard. In the light of this, the present analysis "is concerned with the consistent repetition of particular punctuation marks in, to a broad extent, predictable environments that neatly show when that mark of punctuation was actually used and what its basic purpose was" (Calle-Martín and Miranda-García 2005b: 100).

(16) ¶ also vnderstond þat þer be. 5. maner of whitnesse in vryn. i. þat is bryȝt. and clere moch toward grenesse. and euermore such maner of vryn betokenyth. malencoly. (f. 5v)

c. At phrase level, this symbol sporadically serves to mark off the elements of the phrase, connecting the determiner to the head of the phrase, an adjective to its noun or a preposition to its phrases (Alonso-Almeida 2002: 221–222; Calle-Martín 2004: 416; Calle-Martín and Miranda-García 2005a: 41–42). Instead of an implicit pause therein, the punctus in these cases is conceived as a visual aid to associate the elements of the phrase, thus enabling an appropriate reading of the utterance, as in examples (17–18):

(17) [...] also vryn lacteus somtyme betokenyth. þat. a. man is broste withynne (f. 10v)

(18) [...] yf she be traueyled with. a ffeuer. and haþ not here fflouris it betokenyth deth. (f. 23r)

The punctus is also used with an intra-phrasal function to circumscribe numerals, irrespective of whether they are Roman or Arabic numerals, cardinal and ordinal numbers included. The mark of punctuation is systematically avoided if the numeral is spelled out, as in (19–20):

(19) ¶ also the .i. or þe .2. or þe .3. month þe vryn shall haue smale clowdys withynne. with a white grownde and þe vryn shal be riȝt clere and shynnyng. and þey þat be .4. monthys goyn þer vryn shal be clere red. and þe grownde white shynnyng. auycenna. (f. 40r)

(20) [...] and in þe ffyrste spice of þe etyk. or þe .2. it apere lyke bren. þat hath a lytyl ffloure with him. and /it\ aperyth of þe thryde spice of þe etyk gretter (f. 37v)

1.6.3.2. MS Rylands 1310

Ry presents a more complex system of punctuation, displaying an inventory of seven symbols: the paragraph, the punctus, the virgule, the perioslash, the comma, the colon and the parenthesis. The number of symbols is surely associated with the ongoing process of specialisation of punctuation in eModE (Calle-Martín 2020; also Alonso-Almeida and Ortega-Barrera 2014; Salles-Bernal 2016). Punctuation is historically noted to develop from the rhetorical to the grammatical, from the speaker to the reader, the Renaissance standing out as the transitional period with the adoption of wider syntactic and pragmatic functions to organise the written information and to facilitate the readers' understanding (Lucas 1971: 4; Calle-Martín and Miranda-García 2008: 357; Ronberg 1995: 58). The expression of these syntactic and pragmatic functions eventually resulted in the use of a wider inventory of symbols. This standardisation is elsewhere regarded as a consequence of the introduction of Caxton's printing press in England, the increasing activity of Westminster's Royal Chancery and a growing number of professional scriveners engaged in the writing of all sorts of documents, from guild's records to private letters (Salmon 1999: 15). Notwithstanding, the existence of a received pattern of punctuation among eModE writers cannot be overestimated inasmuch as the inventory and uses of punctuation symbols were usually subject to modifications. Punctuation symbols still preserved overlapping uses, both over time and across text types. All this considered, the functions of marks of punctuation in *Ry* are reproduced in the following sections.

- *The paraph mark*: there are 474 instances of the paraph in the text. When compared with *Hu*, the eModE scribe is less concerned with the use of this mark of punctuation, which is perhaps connected with the growing importance of longer paragraphs in this version. The rendering of longer paragraphs significantly reduces the systematic dependence on this symbol before every single commentary. Notwithstanding its more constrained occurrence, the paraph is here seen to have the same macro-textual function, introducing the authorities' commentaries and acting as a visual aid for the beginning of a new diagnosis of urine. Example (21) reproduces the early Modern version of example (1), where the paraph replicates its late ME use. In addition to this, the paraph is used to highlight important pieces of information, be they a definition or the medicine recommended for the cure of a particular colour of the urine, as in (22):

> (21) ¶ And if it be thik. and inequal it betokenith roring. and hurling and distempering in the body. ev*er*mor in souch party as thow seist it in the vryn*e*: so it is in the body Auic*enna* 4º. ¶ And vryn blac whether it be equal or vnequal. if it be w*ith* a litil body that is litil in quantite sig*nificat* mort*em* ysaac. ¶ Also an vryn that is moch and dark. dym and swart. betokeneth mortificac*io*n than it is more blacker than whan it is of the warissi*ng* of þe feu*er* q*ua*rte*in*. (f. 1r)

> (22) ¶ Medicina ¶ Take scabious herbe benet saug horhound enula campana isop figg*es* licor*is* and boil hem in a galon of water to a potel and vse to drink it often ¶ It*em* Take pou*der* of polipody and aloe Epatik, and medle these together w*ith* sugr*e* and vse it in potage. (f. 9r)

- *The punctus*: there are 834 instances of this mark of punctuation, making it by far the most used symbol in the text. The scribal dependence on this symbol is a crucial testimony to a) the higher need for marking grammatical boundaries; and b) its multiplicity of functions. In eModE, this mark of punctuation is particularly employed to express sentential and clausal relationships as a device to delimit sense-units, in a manner similar to its present-day use. Nevertheless, "the process was not straightforward inasmuch as the period preserved many of its inter-clausal functions until the seventeenth century" (Calle-Martín and Miranda-García 2008: 363). In *Ry*, however, it does not express clausal relations, and the scribe is mostly concerned with rendering sentential boundaries:

a. To mark off the end of a sense-unit, to indicate its boundaries, as shown in example (23):

> (23) ¶ yf the circule be red it tokneth peyn i*n* the forhede. blac tokneth falli*ng* evil. (f. 2v)

b. To connect coordinate sentences, irrespective of the coordinator involved, as in (24–25):

> (24) Take scamony and put it in a per*e*. and rost it. and ete it. (f. 3v)

> (25) THIS CRINOYDES ben caused as furfura saf furfura comyth more of the bladder. But Crinoydes comyth oonly of the membres that be more thik and depe than whan it is of the bladd*er* as it is of the brest and of the sp*irit*uall*is* (f. 18v)

c. To connect subordinate clauses. Nominal clauses are systematically left unpunctuated, the punctus appearing exclusively where there is some intervening material between the matrix verb and the coordinate clause itself, as in (26). Contrary to present-day English practice, adjectival clauses are frequently unpunctuated, regardless of whether there is a restrictive or a non-restrictive relative clause, as shown in (27–28). In adverbial subordination, however, the punctus is a recurrent symbol to connect the main and the subordinate clause, as in examples (29–30), especially in clauses of condition, cause and manner, while the others are unpunctuated. This picture explains the constrained dimension of this symbol if compared with *Hu*, where these relationships were all rendered with a mark of punctuation.

> (26) And therfor Ysodorus saith in the fourth boke of Ethimolog*ies* vj° ca*pitul*o. That Spasmus is the lesse co*n*tractio*un* of partise in the body comyng sodenly in the synows w*ith* houg payn*e* caused of replecio*un* of wiked humours in the synows (f. 13r)

(27) ¶ Blac vrin that is sotel and thy*n*n from the begynnyng of siknesse it betokneth deth*e*. (ff. 2r–2v)

(28) it betokneth a feuer that men cal Sinochus that is a fever engenderd of roten blode in the bodi and veynes. (f. 2v)

(29) ¶ And if it fal down lumpy. as it were whete floure. it tokneth w*ith*holding of her floure*s* Egid*ius* (f. 19r)

(30) Euery blac iposta*sis* is not for to dred. for sumtym it apperith blac because of melancoly (f. 20v)

d. To enumerate items in a series (31):

(31) ¶ And if it cum of the reynes it is pure and litel and sumtym myxt w*ith* thurin and thuryn wil stynk and signifieth the ston. and great siknes. and payn in the bac Ypoc*ras* (f. 17r)

e. To mark off parenthetical constructions (32), i.e. *that is to say, id est,* etc.:

(32) ¶ White vrin and thyn w*ith* smal gravel as it ware chisele and the next vrin befor*e* was white and thik it betokneth nefresis. i*d est.* that is the ston in the raynes Ysaac. (f. 3v)

f. To circumscribe numerals, especially in postposition (33):

(33) ¶ White vrin and thik in the cretik day and namely in the 4. day betokneth a postym*e* behynd the Eris. and after that dethe Ysaac. (f. 5r)

▪ *The colon*: historically derived from the raised period, the colon was already in use in the fourteenth century (Petti 1977: 26). It initially indicated a pause of medium length, but after the introduction of the semicolon at the end of the sixteenth century it evolved as "an indicator of text coherence expressing logically consecutive or adversative relations" (Görlach 1991: 58). The colon is sporadically used in the text to call attention to what follows, as a visual token to draw attention to an important piece of information. In example (34) it highlights that, with such a diagnosis, the patient suffers from *mortification of humours*, but not of the body members.

(34) Also if liuidus color occupi al the vryn*e* or els occupy but part of the vryn*e* the which infectith ov*er* al: it betokneth mortificatio*un* of humores and not of membres (f. 2v)

and stance; and c) to refer to the medical authorities. In (45), the writer introduces an apposition (*with the grace of god*) that is not necessary for the understanding of this diagnosis. In example (46), the parenthesis is used to provide meta-textual material referring back to a similar statement in the treatise. In (47), in turn, it refers to Avicenna as an uroscopic authority in the field in an attempt to demonstrate the scientific endorsement of this particular issue:

> (45) ¶ Ypostasis that is red tokneth long siknes. but (with the grace of god) it is sure./ And if it be temp*er*at red in the begy*n*nin*g* of a siknesse it tokneth that the siknes shal dissolue on the 7 day Ysa*ac*. (f. 20r)

> (46) ¶ And whan it is in the botom (as it is rehersed before) it tokneth payn in the reynes and su*m*tym in the codde w*ith* siknesse in the bladd*er* w*ith* priking in the lonke or nefresi or the tenasmon Ysaac (f. 17r)

> (47) ¶ And (as auic*enna* sayth) if ther aper in thuryn*e* a thyn body moch*e* toward raw silke. and than thattomes be red or rody or smale the colour of the pappis changing ande swelling. (f. 19r)

1.6.4. Emendations

Hu presents the three types of emendations, which include deletion, alteration and insertion (Petti 1977: 29). As far as deletion is concerned, the scribe combines the use of cancellation, obliteration and expunctuation, or even all three together. Cancellation consists in striking through the redundant element(s) with one or more straight lines (48); obliteration means that a word is covered with ink (49), "either by blotting, smudging or completely obscuring the word with cancellation" (Petti 1977: 29); while expunctuation is shown by the dot-underlining of the erroneous letters or words in the text, this becoming frequent in the Latin verses.

Alterations consist in the modification of letters or words by the superimposition or superscription of the correct letter over the deleted one, either by the scribe himself or by a different hand. *Hu* presents different types of alteration, especially in the Latin pieces, showing that the original scribe did have a limited knowledge of that language, as in example (50). Insertions, in turn, are performed directly in the line (interlineation), or in the margin, depending on the length of the insertion, whether they be words, phrases or clauses, as shown in (51). Insertions in *Hu* are frequently provided in the marginalia, and the caret (^) indicates the point at which the fragment is to be inserted (Petti 1977: 29). Insertions are either by the scribe himself or by later scribes, where a change in the handwriting is easily noticed.

(48) also blak vryn is causyd ~~is causyd~~ of. iij thyngys. i. because of adustion. 2. because of mortificac*io*n. 3. or w*ith* nig*er* hum*our*. i*d est*. Malencoly. (f. 1v)

(49) and yelwe spwme ~~spwma~~ in a wo*m*man betoken*yth* rete*n*cion of fflouris (f. 23v)

(50) Si forma*m* causon in febre viror/i\s ad/o\ptat. (f. 27v)

(51) ¶ also Cin*er*is ben asshys yf þey aper*e* in þe vryn /and p*ri*ncipally it betoken*yth* wasty*n*g of the lu*n*gg*is*. *and* consu*m*pc*io*n of þe body\. it betokenyth syknes. *and* dissesys beneth forth as fic*us*. or þe enrawdys. and þe tetis or bigg*us* of þe emrawdys to swoln. Egidi*us*. (f. 40v)

The early modern version of the text, on the other hand, is more limited in terms of the number and typology of emendation techniques, as it stands out for being a more elaborated copy than its mediaeval counterpart. The scribal concern about the external appearance of this version justifies, for instance, the absence of alterations in the witness. The other emendation techniques are, however, more sporadically employed. Deletion is elsewhere performed through the cancelling of the unnecessary item(s), either in black or red ink, the latter preferentially when the deleted element is a longer statement. Insertions are in all cases rendered on the line of writing made by the scribe himself as a result of an erroneous omission of a few words during the writing process. (52) reproduces both a scribal deletion and insertion.

(52) ¶ And /suche\ maner vryn betokneth ever indigestio*u*n of homowrs in the body Ysaac. ¶ Vnderstonde the white vrin and thyn*e* is indigestion and defaute of ~~vn~~kindly hete. and these be the toknes therof. (f. 3r)

1.6.5. Abbreviations

It was a common practice in handwritten documents to abbreviate words in foreign languages such as Latin, French or Greek, and this habit was eventually transferred to the vernacular, where a large number of abbreviations are found (Tannenbaum 1930: 119). Based on the Latin tradition, scribes incorporated the classical methods of abbreviation into their compositions (Tannenbaum 1930: 119). *Hu*, as a fifteenth-century composition, displays a higher number of abbreviations than its eModE counterpart. Both witnesses, however, present the same abbreviation techniques, with instances of contraction, suspension, brevigraphs and superscript letters.

a. Contraction is one of the commonest methods of abbreviation in historical manuscripts, consisting in the omission of one or more letters within a word as a substitute for the letters <m>, <n>, <u> and <i>, the latter exclusively in the -ion suffix (Calle-Martín and Miranda-García 2012: 39). The contractions were indicated by means of the bar, which was the most frequent symbol for this kind of abbreviation (Petti 1977: 22). In *Hu*, this method was employed to omit one single letter within the word, as in Figs 5–6 below.

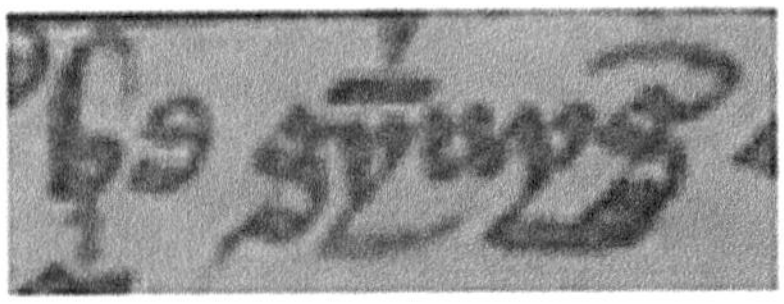

Fig. 5. begyn*nyng* (f. 3v)

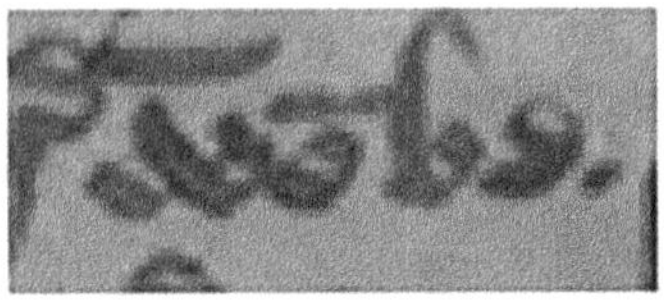

Fig. 6. wo*m*be (f. 5v)

b. Curtailment, also termed suspension, was the shortening of the end of the word by one or more letters (Tannenbaum 1930: 124). The abbreviation was occasionally marked with a horizontal bar above the terminal part of the word, as in Figure 7.

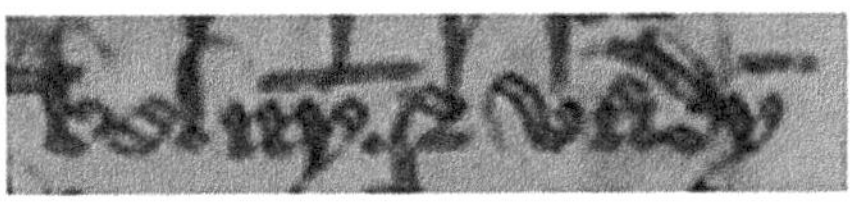

Fig. 7. bolny*n* *and* va*n*dy*n*

c. Brevigraphs consist in the use of special signs to contract a number of frequently occurring syllables, particularly at the beginning and at the end of a word. Medial positions, albeit sporadic, become less frequent from the fifteenth century (Calle-Martín and Miranda-García 2012: 40) Even though the inventory of brevigraphs was mostly adapted from Latinate texts, some others progressively acquired vernacular uses. Thus, both *Hu* and *Ry* display the typical set of brevigraphs found in fifteenth- and sixteenth-century handwritten documents, the list including the <s> and the <r> clusters. The former includes the clusters <er> (i.e. an ascending flourished stroke curved leftwards) and <ur> (i.e. a superscript letter <a>), as in feu*er*, wat*er*, sauo*ur*, colo*ur*, etc. The latter displays the clusters <par>/<per> (i.e. a straight bar through the stem), the cluster <pro> (i.e. the letter <p> with a curved stroke through the descender), as in p*ar*t, p*er*el, p*ro*longacio*u*n, etc.

d. Superscript letters were used to omit one or more letters at the end of the word, and they were placed above the line to indicate the omission. This abbreviation technique could be applied to all words and the number of omitted letters could vary according to the scribe. The following superscript letters are found in *Hu*: w^{t} > w*it*h, þ^{t} > þ*a*t, betoken^{t} > betoken*yth*, and the like.

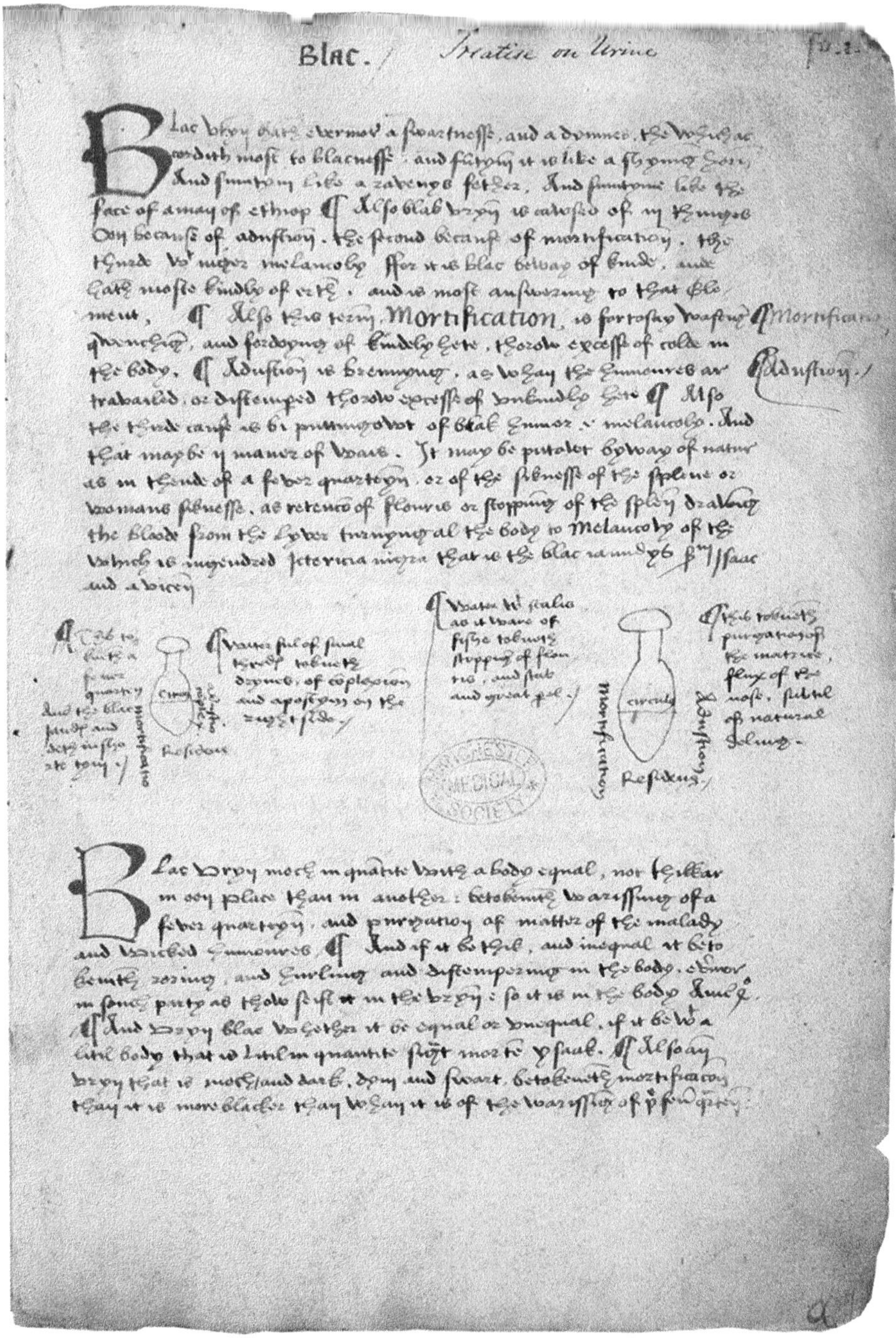

Plate 3. MS Rylands 1310 (f. 1r)

2. Text

2.1. Editorial conventions

This work stems from the project entitled *The Málaga Corpus of Early English Scientific Prose*, which pursues the semi-diplomatic edition of hitherto unedited late Middle English and early Modern English scientific prose published online together with their manuscript originals (covering the historical period 1300–1700). These editions eventually serve as the input for the compilation of a tagged corpus of late Middle English and Early Modern English scientific prose. The late Middle English and the early Modern English components of the corpus, together with the electronic editions, can be freely accessed at http://hunter.uma.es and http://modernmss.uma.es.

This chapter offers the synoptic edition of the English vernacular versions of *De judiciis urinarum*, preserved in two witnesses from the early fifteenth and sixteenth centuries, respectively. The edition has been conceived as a textual resource for academic scholarship in different disciplines: not only Historical Linguistics but also Codicology, Palaeography and the History of Medicine. For this reason, the rationale of a *semi-diplomatic edition* has been adopted so as to provide an accurate reproduction of the sources. The editorial conservatism in a synoptic edition is a desideratum in cases where there are different versions of the same text, thus serving "the compromise between respecting the qualities of the textual versions [...] and making the texts and their differences adequately available to the modern reader" (Tronch 2002: 72).

The transcription is rendered in different font sizes for a better organisation of the material. The Latin verses in *Hu* are reproduced in a smaller size as a visual indication to the reader of the beginning of a new section. Some sections include drawings of urine flasks accompanied by text discussing the most significant illnesses related to that particular urine colour. This material has also been reproduced in a smaller size in view of its appearance in the witnesses, rendered with a more compact typeface as a result of the limited space for writing because of the presence of the urine flasks.

Our transcription is therefore graphemic, to keep the reader as close as possible to the manuscript versions, and complies with the following guidelines, partially adapted from Petti (1977: 24–35). The spelling,[1] capitalisation, punctuation and word division of the original manuscript have been retained in the edition. Abbreviations have been expanded with the supplied letter(s) italicised.[2] Superior letters are lowered to the line, as in w^{t} > w*it*h or þ^{e} > þe. Insertions have been rendered in their proper sequence in the body of the text, noted with the use of / \ when the material is inserted above the line and // \\ if in the margin.

The edition is accompanied by three apparatuses. The first is used for scribal corrections, where cancellations (*cancel.*), obliterations (*oblit.*), expunctuations (*exp.*), deletions (*del.*) and repetitions (*rep.*) have been supplied. The second contains the marginal information, noting whether it appears in the external margin (*ext. marg.*), the internal margin (*int. marg.*), the top margin (*top. marg.*) or the bottom margin (*bot. marg.*). In the particular case of *Hu*, the apparatus also incorporates the modifications by a later scribe, which become particularly frequent in the Latin pieces. These modifications may be insertions (*ins.*), corrections by expunctuation (*corr. by exp.*) or by cancellation (*corr. by cancel.*) or just a change of word order (*transp.*). The exact position of these changes – whether they are written above (*suprascr.*) or below the line (*subscr.*) – is also noted in the apparatus. The third apparatus is used to clarify the editorial interpretation of some obscure readings and odd spellings of the Latin excerpts in *Hu*.

Finally, the edition includes the translation of the Latin material from Giles de Corbeil's *Carmen de urinis* housed in the Hunterian witness. Originally written in verse, the Latin original is a dense mnemonic text with a difficult translation, more often than not requiring the clarification of obscure and omitted senses. For convenience, a direct translation is here proposed to provide the reader with an accurate rendering of the Latin original, in which lineation has also been preserved to facilitate cross-referencing between the Latin and its present-day English versions. Square brackets are used to provide the senses that need to be supplied for the correct understanding of the original, while inverted commas serve to render the translation of Latin into Middle English in the manuscript witness. Punctuation, in turn, is modernised in view of the absence of marks of punctuation in the original.

1 The different renderings of a same consonant, however, have been normalised, particularly in the case of the letter <s>, represented by means of the long <s> and the eight-shaped <s> in *Hu*.

2 Superfluous brevigraphs and otiose flourishes, in turn, have been ignored.

MS Hunter 328

.Ihc.

f. 1r Ego magist*er* Ioh*an*nes Arderon /hoc\ opusculu*m* co*m*posui de Iudicijs Vrina*rum* p*er* colores & contenta s*ecundum* Iudiciu*m* Egidij. & ypoc*ras*. wa/l\t*erius*. Gilbert*us*. Gor*dianus*. Ioh*an*nes de s*anto* Amando. ysaac. Auicen*na*. theophil*us*. Galyen. Galt*erius*. & tholome*us*. in medicina. & medicini d*omi*n*i* regis illustrissi p*r*incipis henrici quarti cui*us* a*ni*m*e* p*ro*piciet*ur* deus. Amen.

. de. nigra. vrina. capitulu*m*. p*ri*mu*m*.
Nigrior vrine faciens inco*m*moda febris.
Quartane soluit. morte*m* po*r*tendit adurit.
Si nig*er* ad fu*n*du*m* residens se repr/i\mit humor.
Matrix pu/r\gat*ur* multi sentina fluoris.
In febre fert mortis nig*ra*. fetida pauca
Vecise vicio pros*us* renu*mque* remoto
Multa die cretico q*uam* nig*raque* pendula nubes.
Largi*us* obfuscat sedimenq*ue* natalie turbat.
Aurib*us* oppressis turbata pauce s/o\poris.
Sang*ui*neu*m* fluxu*m* sig*na*t de nare futuru*m*.
Quod si signa mali co*n*currat sine salutis.
Iudic*i*o mortis da*m*pnat. *vel*. liberat egru*m*.
*con*grua mixture cu*m* spisso federa *ser*uans.
Subtilis coitu*m* refugit nigredo liquoris.
Vt tenue*m* tollerat *qui* no*n* sibi *con*colore heret.
Impetrat event*us* cas*usque* facit violent*us*.
Non obstrusa paru*m* deducc*i*o clausa via*rum*.
Bis deni vrina*m* possu*n*t variare colores.
Quos ex hijs scriptis poteris p*er*pend*er*e formis.

Also þu shalt und*er*stonde and knowe þ*a*t blak uryn haþ eu*er* mor*e* a swartnesse *and* a dy*n*nesse the wech acordyth inofte to blaknesse. and

3 Arderon] *cancel.* hoc | **7** wa/l\terius] *cancel.* Gilis | **22** nigraque] *exp. que* | **24** s/o\poris] *exp.* a. MS saporis | **26** mali] *exp. concur*rat | **28** congrua] *cancel. uel* | **34** hijs] *cancel.* sprit*is*

2 Ihc] *top. marg.* Michael | **16** faciens] *corr. by exp.* facies *m.r.* | **19** fluoris] *corr. by exp. and suprascr.* tumoris *m.r.* | **20** febre] *ext. marg.* a paciente cum membre in febre acute. | mortis] *ins. by suprascr.* signu*m* *m.r.* | **22** nigraque] *corr. by exp.* and *suprascr.* nigra /et\ *m.r.* | **23** natalie] *ins. by suprascr.* nata/bi\lie *m.r.* | **24** s/o\poris] *corr. by exp.* and *suprascr.* s/o\poris *m.r.* | **26** concurrat] *corr. by exp.* //co*n*curra*n*t\\ | **30** tollerat] *corr. by exp. and suprascr.* toller/e\t *m.r.* | concolore] *corr. by cancel.* concolor *m.r.* | **32** obstrusa] *corr. by exp. and suprascr.* obuclusa *m.r.*

MS Rylands 1310

Blac. f. 1r

Blac vryn hath evermor*e* a swartnesse. and a dymnes. the which accordith most to blacnesse. and su*m*tym*e* it is like a shyni*n*g horn*e* And sumtym like a ravenys fether. And sumtyme like the face of a man of ethiop ¶ Also blak vryn*e* is cawsed of iij thinges Oon because of adustion. the second because of mortification. the thirde w*ith* niger melancoly ffor it is blac be way of kinde. ande hath moste kindly of erth. and is most answering to that Element. ¶ Also this term. mortification. is for to say wasti*n*g qwenchi*n*g. and fordoyng of kindely

4 Blac] *top marg.* Treatise on Urine *m.r.* | **13** mortification] *ext. marg.* ¶ mortificacio*n*

downward it betoken*yth* lyff. and it be co*ntrar*y it is deth. and whan it is so blak. stynkyng. *and* ffatty it betoken*yth* sykenes i*n* þe bladd*er*. and in þe reynes. and it betoknyt mortifycac*io*n of rotyn hum*er*s. and meltyng of nature w*ith* stoppyng of þe lyu*er*. throutt hote scaldyng hum*er*s. and betoken*ith* grete p*er*el. auic*enna*. 4°. *and* Galyen.

¶ also blak vryn in a ffeu*er* w*ith* blak ypostasys nat in the botom but upward in þe myddys. *and* no slepe. w*ith* deyffhed and it betoken*yth* þat þe maledy wyll laste long. and if he blede at the nose. sig*nifica*t salute*m*. ysaac.

¶ also blak vryn in a brenyng feu*er*. *and* grevance i*n* þe hed w*ith* anguish. and ravyng. and faylyng of mynde it betokenyth warysshyng of sykenes w*ith* bledyng at þe nose. anamely in wo*m*men þat han had her*e* fflourys. auic*enna*. pri*mo*.

¶ also blak vryn. and þycke in an agu betoken*yth* þe krampe and if he /have\ ravyng. *and* wlatyng it betoken*yth* deth. ysaac.

¶ also vryn blak as blood þ*at* is swartt. *and* dy*m*me in a phiresys betokenyth deth. ysaac.

¶ also an vryn blak i*n* an agu and þe ypostasys be not hooll. but in dyu*er*se plottys. *and* it change ofte his colo*ur* it betokenyth deth. Egidi*us*.

¶ also an vryn blak. *and* stynkyng. and swetyng in the nethyr partyes. it betokenyth. deth. auic*enna*.

¶ also black vryn moste lyke to citryne. or glauke colour w*ith* ypostasis betoken*yth* eu*er* þ*at* red. coler. is aduste. and brenny*n*g wythynne. and þe black Iawndys. w*ith*
f. 3r hevynesse. *and* anguish. | and peyne in þe hed *and* strong sauo*ur*. *secundu*m. ysaaç. & auic*ena*. pri*mo*.

¶ Galyen seyth þ*at* in tyme of pestylence a black vryn w*ith* good signes. sig*nifica*t salute*m*. and be *contr*ary it is deth. Eu*er* þe more thycker þ*at* vryn is the thy*n*ner the //wersse\\ but in bothe is p*er*el. auic*enna*. pri*mo*. &. 2°. 4°. ff. 2°.

157 the] *rep.* þe | 192 is] *cancel.* þe mor*e* p*er*el

¶ Also blac vryn in a brenny*ng* fever and greuaunce in the hede of anguish and raving and failing of mynde it be/to\kenith warisshing of siknesse w*ith* bleding at the nose. and namly in wy*m*men that hath had her flour*is* Auic*enna* p*rimo*.

¶ Blac vryn and thik in an agw betokenith the cra*m*pe / and if he haue raving and wlating it betokenith deth Ysaac

¶ Vrin blac as blood that is swart and dy*m*me in a pleure*sis* betokenith deth. Ysaac.

¶ Blac vryn in an agw. and the ypostasis be not hole but in diuerse plottis and it chaunge ofte his colour it betokenith deth. Egidius.

¶ Vrin blac and stinkinge and swete in the nether p*ar*ties it betokenith deth. Auicen*na*.

¶ Blac vrin most like to citrin or f. 2r
glauce colour w*ith* yposta*sis* betokeneth ever the red colour is adust and bre*nni*ng w*ith*in and the blac iaundes w*ith* hevynes. and angwish and payn in the hede and strong sauo*ur* *secundu*m isaac and auic*enna* p*rimo*

¶ Galen saith that in tyme of pestilens a blac vrin w*ith* good synis sig*nifica*t salute*m*. and it be contrary it is deth Euer the mor thikker that vryn is the thynner the worse but in both is p*er*el Auic*enna* p*rimo* 24 ff 2°.

¶ And Gualteri*us* seith 2° pronostic*es* co*n*tra 22. that vrin shewith ever of grose humoures co*n*sum*p*tion made be adustion and the cra*m*p thorow drawing and driy*n*g of senows

¶ Blac vrin in which is sedimen gatherd and hanging blac and rownd w*ith* an evil sauo*ur* betokenith apostem vnder the right side and the cramp swet and dethe auic*ena* 4

¶ Blac vryn sotel and litil pessima est Ysaac Ypoc*ras* saith that in tym of pestilence betokenith adustion of humores. and the vryn be blak. and also if it be sotel w*ith* a litil feu*er* it

127 wymmen] *cancel.* whan | 154 the[1]] *cancel.* mor

¶ and Galt*er*ius seyth. 2º. p*ro*nosticis *contra*. 32. þ*a*t g*ro*se vryn shew*yth* eu*er* of g*ro*se hum*er*is. co*nsum*pc*i*on causyd by adustion. and the krampe throuh drawyng. and dryyng of senuys.

¶ also an vryn black in þe wech is sedymen gaderyd *and* hangyng black *and* rownde w*ith* an evyl sauo*ur* betokenyth a postym vnd*er* þe ryȝt syde. *and* þe krampe. swett. *and* deþ. auic*enn*a. 4º.

¶ also black vryn. sotyl and lytel. pessi*m*a e*st*. ysaac. ypocras. seyth þ*a*t in tyme of pestylence betokenyth adustion of hum*er*is. and þe vryn be black. and also yf it be sotyl w*ith* a liȝtt ffeu*er* it betokenyth grete anguysh. anamely of wo*m*menys syknes. and þe Emrawdys. ysaac.

¶ also black vryn. w*ith* peyne. *and* anguysh in þe hed wyth stoppyng of breth. and alyenac*i*on of mynde betokenyth g*re*te plente of wo*m*me*n*nys fflourys. s*ecundu*m. ysaac.

¶ and black vryn in a man w*ith* a sharpe feu*er*. shortt breth *and* swett on þe hed. þe necke. or þe back. pessi*m*a e*st*. s*ecundu*m**.** ysaac. & theo*p*hil*us*. ¶ and in wo*m*men it betokenyth grete helthe. auic*enn*a. 4º. and aft*er* t*ra*velyng of chyld it betoken*yth* þe crampe. black vryn bothe in man. and in wo*m*man it is wyckyd. but it is worsse *and* /more\ susspecte i*n* men. ysaac. 2º. p*ro*nostic*is*. & *contra*. 33º.

¶ and it be black. *and* moch it is deth. s*ecundu*m. ysaac. and it be black. and vyscouse. w*ith* swetyng. and peyne in þe ryȝt syde. betokenyth deth. co*n*stantyn*us*. 7º. pan*tegni*. & v*er*asis. ixº.

¶ and if it pyssyd black. or red. and com throuh drynkyng of wyn. þe*ry*nne is no drede. s*ecundu*m. auic*enna*. p*ri*mo.

¶ and black vryn com in þe
f. 3v begy*n*nyng of a sykenes wyth | drede. and abydyth so tyl þe. 7. day. *and* þan comyth a good colo*ur* w*ith* white ypostatis. it betokenyth brekyng of þe maledy. but if þ*er* com /no\ good signes. but peyne. *and* shortte breth swett on þe membrys vpward. *and*

betokenith great angwish and namely of womans sikness and the emeraudis Ysaac.

¶ Blac vryn w*ith* payn and angwish in the hed w*ith* stopping of breth. and alienation of mynd betokenyth great plenti of womans flour*is* s*ecundu*m Ysaac

¶ Blac vryn in a man w*ith* a sharp feuer shorte breth and swete of the hede the nek or the bac pessima e*st* Ysaac. theophil*us*. And in woman it betokeneth great helth Auic*enna* 4º and after travaling of child it betokneth cramp / blac vryn both in man and woma*n* it is wiked. but it is worse and more suspecte in man Ysaac 2 pronostic*es* & *contra* 33º.

¶ Blac and moch it is deth ysaac and it be blac and viscouse w*ith* sweting and payn in the right side it betokneth deth Constantin*us* 7º. pan*tegni* & v*er*asis ixº./

¶ And if it pissid blac or red and cum thorow drynkyng of wyn ther is no drede. Auic*enna* p*ri*mo.

¶ Blac vryn co*m* in the beginnyng of a siknesse w*ith* drede and abidith so til the seventh day and than cu*m*myth good colour w*ith* white ypostasis it betoknyth breking of the maledy but if ther cum no good synes but payn and short breth swet on thi membres vpward and alienation of mynde non appetite it betokeneth deth ysaac

¶ Blac vryn if gren went before it betoknyth great adustion of blood Egidius. and it betokneth melancoly auic*enna* p*ri*mo

¶ Blac vrin and thik w*ith* ypostasis famouse and fatty and litil stynking w*ith*out payn in the bac / or the bladder it betokneth great adustion and deth ¶ And if he have payn in the reynes it betoknyth peyn or a postom broke in the reynes Walterius

¶ And blac colour change often and haue a blac cloude w*ith* the frenesy sig*nifica*t mortem Ioa*n*nes de s*anct*o amando

187 is[1]] *cancel.* wyk

alyenac*i*on of mynde. noon appetite it betokenyth deth. *secundum* ysaac

¶ also black vryn if grene wentte before it betoken*yth* grete adustyon. of blood. s*ecundu*m. Egidiu*m*. & sig*nifica*t mel*anco*liam. auic*enna*. p*rim*o.

¶ Vryn þ*a*t is black. *and* thycke. *and* w*ith* ypostasys ffamose. *and* ffatty. and lytel. sty*n*kyng. w*ith*out peyne i*n* þe back or þe bladd*er* it betoke grete adustyon. *and* deth. //¶\\ and if he haue peyne in þe reynes it betokenyth peyne. *and* a postym broke in þe reynys. walterius.

¶ and black colo*ur* chong oftyn. *and* haue a black clowde w*ith* þe frenesy. sig*nifica*t morte*m*. s*ecundu*m. Ioh*an*em. de s*ancto* amando.

¶ Black vryn þ*a*t is sotyl *and* thy*n*ne f/r\om þe begy*nn*y*n*g of syknes it betokenyth deth. co*n*stanti*nus*. 7º. pantegn*i*.

Take Celidonie. sp*er*macete. triacle. *conser*ua rosaru*m*. and drynke it w*ith* white wyne. &c.

. contra vim mortis no*n* est medicamen in ortis.
. de liuida vrina cui*us* color est ut color plu*m*bi.
liuida si fuerit liuor. *v*el. perticulares.
Vrine varias liuoris collige causas.
Vel tota *uel* erit p*er* totu*m* liuida menbris.
aut membri monst*rat* humore*m* mortificari.
¶ aut sursu*m* liuuis variis accomoda causis.
P*aruus* emitrite*us* medi*us* morb*usque* medi*us* caduc*us*.
alchites sinoc*us* vene ruptura catarr*us*.
Strangurie laps*us* mat*ri*cis passio flux*us*.
Coste pulmonis viciu*m* dolor articularis.
Consuptiua ptisis vix extincta caloris.
Sint tibi liuoris cause quas collige signis.
Paucula vix iunta liuens oleagina morte*m*.
Strangu*r*ia*m* monst*rat* liuida pauca frequens.
f. 4r liuor cu*m* gra*n*is se iunctis at*que* minutis.

¶ Blac vrin that is sotel and thyn from | the begynnyng of siknesse it betokneth deth. Constantin*us* 7º pantegn*i*

¶ MEDICINA

¶ Take Celode*in* sp*er*macete. triacle. conserua rosaru*m*. and drink it w*ith* whighte wyn &c ¶ Contra vim mortis no*n* est medicamen in ortis

---

273 Take] *ext. marg.* medicina | **276** contra] *ext. marg.* vnde v*ersus* | **277** liuida] *ext. marg.* bloo col*our* | **278** perticulares] *corr. by cancel.* perticularis *m.r.* | **279** Vrine] *ext. marg.* ca*pitulum* s*ecundum* | **280** tota uel] *corr. by exp. and suprascr.* totalis *m.r.* | **282** liuuis] *corr. by exp. and suprascr.* liuens *m.r.* | **283** morbusque medius] *transp.* medi*us* morb*usque m.r.* | **287** vix] *corr. by exp. and suprascr.* vis *m.r.* | **288** signis] *corr. by exp. and suprascr.* sanguis *m.r.* | **289** iunta] *corr. by exp. and suprascr.* iuncta *m.r.*

---

289 Paucula…mortem] A change of metre from hexameters to elegiacs

Constant*er* loquit*ur* spir*itu*ale malu*m*.
Liuiditas athomosa malu*m* p*ro*bat articulo*rum*
Est q*uoque* Rewmatici iu*n*cta sida mali.
Vertebru*m* si mat*rix* oppressit aut diafragma.
Inficit vrine liuid*us* ora color

Bloo colo*ur*. or ledy. or wan colo*ur*. all is on. lyke toward white. *and* black. havyng oneþys more of þe black þan of þe white. somtyme it betokenyth. adustyon. and som tyme Mortifycac*i*on. Whan it aperyth w*ith* a grenesse it betoken*yth* adustyon / and if þ*er* apere noo*n* it betokenyt Mortifycac*i*on. *secundu*m. theophilu*m*. & Egidiu*m*.

Also yf liuid*us* colo*ur* ocupye all þe vryne. or ell*es* ocupy but a p*ar*t of þe vryn þe wech enfectyth ou*er* all it betoken*yth* mortificac*i*on of hum*er*is. and nat of me*m*brys // and it be thicke benethe *and* not bloo nor wan above. *and* cler*e*. and þe enfecc*i*on goon awey. þan it betoken*yth*. mortifycac*i*on bothe of hum*er*is. and of me*m*brys. Gilb*ertus*. *libro*. *primo*.

Also a bloo vryn w*ith* a grene c*er*kyl. betokenyth þe fallyng evyl./ and these ben þe names þ*er*of. Epilencia. analempcia. Cathalempcia. morbus caduc*us*. morbus councialis. pedicon. Ierariolon. & Ira dei. In this maledy allwey þe me*m*brys of lyff ben co*n*fecte þrouh cold. an/d\ they ben dul *and* feyntt. and febyl. *and* þ*a*t betokenyth eu*er* the bloo cerkyl. *secundu*m. walt*er*iu*m*.

. ledy. colour.
¶ Epilencia *and* brekyng of me*m*brys. þe ffeu*er* t*er*cian. hard to make wat*er*. *and* þe fflourys. yf the c*er*kyl be red it betokenyth peyne i*n* þe forhed. and if it black it betokenyth the fally*ng* evyl. *secundu*m. Auicenna. 4°.

f. 4v ¶ also bloo colour betokenyth the hote dropsy. i*d est*. alchites and it betokenyth a ffeu*er* þ*a*t men calle Synocus. þ*a*t is a ffeu*er* engendryd of rottyn blood in þe body. *and* i*n* þe

¶ Inficit urine Liuidus ora color./

Bloo color or ledy or wan colour al is on like towarde white and blac having onethis more of the blac than of the white a grenesse it betokneth adustio*un*. And if ther appere non it betoknyth mortification *secundu*m theophilu*m* and Egidiu*m*.

Also if liuidus color occupi al the vryn or els occupy but part of the vryn the which infectith ov*er* al: it betokneth mortification of humores and not of membres and it be thik beneth and not blo nor wan above and clere and the infection gon away than it betokneth mortification both of humoures and of membres. Gilbert*us* *libro* p*rimo*

Blo vryn w*ith* a grene cerkil betokneth the falling evil. and these be the names therof Epilencia. Analemptia. Catalemptia. morb*us* caduc*us*. morbus countialis. pedicon. Ierariolon. et ira dei. In these maledy alwai the membres of lif be enfected thorow colde. and the{y} ben dul. and feynt. and feble ¶ And that betokneth ever the blo circule secu*n*du*m* Walteriu*m* /

¶ Epilentia and breking of membres. the feuer tercian. hard to make water and flour*is*. ¶ yf the circule be red it tokneth peyn i*n* the forhede. blac tokneth falli*ng* evil.

¶ Blo colour betokneth thote dropsey. i*d est*. alchites. and it betokneth a feuer that men cal Sinochus that is a fever engenderd of roten blode in the bodi and veynes. Tholome*us* and Gilbert*us* in Libro 7° /

¶ Vrin Liuidus betokneth ther be veynes broken in the lendys. and a revmatik flux distilling from thede to the lunges. and peyn and akith vnd*er*

313 enfeccion] *cancel.* d | **335** it] *cancel.* be

293 articulorum] *corr. by exp. and suprascr.* articu/lare\ *m.r.* | **294** iuncta] *corr. by exp.* //nu*n*cia\\ *m.r.* | **319** Epilencia] *ext. marg.* Epilencia

294 sida] Opaque word in this context, perhaps *signa* or *sigla*

238 mortification] *oblit.* both of humours and of membres | **245** above] *cancel.* bb. MS a~~bb~~bove

272 lendys] *ext. marg.* lend*ys*

¶ also vnd*er*stond þ*a*t white vryn. and thynne. is indigestyon. and defaute of kyndly hete. and these ben the tokenys þ*er*of. þ*er* is moche wynde in þe body. and bolny*ng*. and acthe in sydes. and swellyng i*n* þe wo*m*be. *and* flownesse. *and* dulnesse. hevynes in þe body. *and* i*n* þe armys *and* i*n* þe leggys. and in all þe body. and ayens þe wytt*is*. and ayens the movyng of þe soule. and Evyl dysposysc*i*on in þe hed anamely in þe lyffte halff. s*ecundu*m. Egidiu*m*.

¶ also vnd*er*stond þ*a*t þ*er* be. 3. man*er* of whitnesse in vryn. i. þ*a*t is bryȝt. *and* clere moch toward grenesse. and eu*er*more such man*er* of vryn betoken*yth*. malencoly. and. pest*ylence* ¶ The. 2. it is somdel bryȝt but þ*a*t is but lytel. somwhat toward rednesse. and in as moch as it is lesse bryȝtt þe body þ*er*of haþ more of thycknesse. þan it betokenyth. Colr*e*. drenchyd in fflewm. and is ou*er*com w*ith* excesse of fflewm. 3. man*er* of vryn þ*a*t is whitte and haþ noo*n* of þese *con*dicions. befor*e* seyd eu*er*more fflewm. and it haue neþ*er* of grenesse nor of rednesse. s*ecundu*m. Egidiu*m*. & Ioh*an*em. d*e*. s*ancto*. a*mando*.

. white. colour.

¶ the wastyng of þe splen. dropsy. ston. wodnes. schaffyng of þe lyu*er*. Emrawdys. stoppy*ng* of þe fflor*is*. white g*ra*vel betokenyth þe ston i*n* þe bladd*er*. black g*ra*vel sig*nifica*t peyne i*n* þe le*n*dys *and* betwyn the kydneys.

f. 6r ¶ also white vryn at þe begy*n*nyng of syknesse. *and* long tyme lastyng w*ith* a man*er* of blohed in þe ou*er* par*t*y of the vryn it betoken*yth*. a syknesse þ*a*t is callyd. yposarca. þ*a*t is þe cold dropsy þ*e* wech is engendryd of salt fflewm. ysaac.

¶ also white vryn. and thy*n*ne. *and* moch in quantyte betoken*yth* excesse of mete. and drynke. Egidi*us*.

¶ also white vryn *and* thy*n*ne w*ith* smal g*ra*uel as it wer*e* chysel. and þe next vryn before was white. *and* thycke. it betokenyth. nefresys. þ*a*t is þe ston in þe reynes. ysaac.

461 moch] *cancel. and exp.* moch | **468** it] *cancel.* an

483 dropsy] *ext. marg.* þe d*ro*psy

Ther is moch wind in the body. and bolnyng. and ach in the the sydes and swelling in the wombe. and flownes dulnes and hevines in the body. and in tharmes. and in the legges | and in al f. 3v
the body and aȝens the witt*is* and ayens the moving of the soule. and evil disposition in thede and namely in the lifte half s*ecundu*m Egidiu*m*

¶ Vnderstond also that ther be ij maner of whitnes in vryn, oon that is bright and clere moche toward grenesse *and* euermor such man*er* vryn betokneth melancoly and pest*ilens*. The second it is sumdele bright but that is but litil. and su*m*what toward rednes and in as moch as it is les bright the body therof have mor of thiknes than it betokneth Coler dre*n*ched in flewm. and is ov*er*cu*m* with excesse of flewm. 3 man*er* of vryn that is white and hath non of these condicions beforsaid euermore flewme and it hath nether of grenes nor of rednesse Egid*ius* & Io*h*an*es*.

¶ wasting of the splen. dropsi. ston. wodnesse chafing of the lyuer. Emeraud*is*. stopi*ng* of the flour*is*. ¶ white g*ra*uel. the ston i*n* the bladd*er* blac, peyn in the lend*is*. and betwen the kidnesse./

¶ White vrin at the begy*n*ni*ng* of siknesse and long tym lasting w*ith* a maner of blohed in the over part of the vryn it betokneth {a siknesse þ*a*t is} called iposarcha that is the cold dropsey. the which is engendred of salt flewm. Ysaac.

¶ White vryn and thyn and moch in qua*n*tite betokneth excesse of mete and drink Egidi*us*

¶ White vrin and thyn w*ith* smal gravel as it ware chisell and the next vrin befor was white and thik it betokneth nefresis. i*d est*. that is the ston in the raynes Ysaac.

¶ Also and the vrin be first thik and afterward white and thik it betokneth the ston in the raynes ysaac./

¶ An vrin white and thyn betokneth the ilyca passion w*ith* hurling

403 thyn] *cancel.* and | **404** the] *eras.* iliaca

¶ also and þe vryn be fyrste thycke. *and* affte*r*ward white and thicke. betokenyth þe ston i*n* þe reynes. ysaac.

¶ also an vryn white *and* thy*n*ne. betokenyth þe ylica pasio w*ith* hurlyng. gnawyng. *and* shetyng i*n* þe guttys. ysaac.

¶ also vryn þ*at* white. *and* thy*n*ne. and moch in quantyte w*ith* smale. *and* long resoluc*io*ns. as it is oþ*er*whyle in water þ*at* fflesh is sodyn y*n*ne betokenyth þe passyon þ*at* is callyd. dyabetes. þ*at* is oue*r*mesur of makyng of wat*er*. and this maledy comyth somtyme of dystemp*er* of hete i*n* þe reynes. and somtyme by excesse of lechery. and somtyme of t*ra*velyng. re*n*ny*n*g or skkyppyng. vn*de* ypoc*ras*. & ysaac.

¶ also an vryn white *and* thy*n*ne. *and* somwhat ȝelwyshe. or g*r*enysh. *and* bryȝtt it betokenyth a sykenes þ*at* is callyd scotomia. *and* vertigo. þ*at* is whan on tu*r*nyth þe eyes. and thynkyth þ*at* all þe world or þe house tu*r*nyth. abowte hym. and yf it com in hervest it betokenyth. a q*ua*rteyn or ellys a cotidyan cauȝt throwh. fflewm. *and* male*n*coly. ysaac. and also thr/o\uh. fflewm vitres. auic*enna*. 4º. //¶\\ and bycause of malencoly hume*r*s in þe body styeng up i*n*to þe hed *and* stoppyng þ*er*. *secundum*. tholome*us*. & Egid*ium*./

¶ also white vryn. *and* /thy*n*ne of\ a chyld. betokenyth. coldnesse of the lyu*er*. *secundu*m. ysaac.

f. 6v ¶ also white colo*ur*. *and* thy*n*ne w*ith* hakyng. *and* pryckyng. and hevynesse abowte þe spawdys. *and* þe shuldrys. *and* þe necke anamely yf he haue greynes vnd*er* þe c*er*kyl. betokenyth a syknes þ*at* is Callyd. lyppotomia. *id est*. Syncopys. or þe Chy*n*cok al is on. *secundu*m**.** Walt*erius*. & Egidiu*m*.

¶ also white vryn. and thy*n*ne i*n* þe day þ*at* þe pacyent haþ his acesse it betoken*yth* a very quarteyn causyd of kynd malencoly. but on þe next day it shuld be pale or subpale. *and* on þe. thryde day. or þ*e*. 4te. day it shulde be wihte. or ȝelwe. and þan it shal loke blackysh. *and* thyck w*ith* moch

518 world] cancel. t*u*ry

gnawing and sheti*n*g in the gutt*is* Ysaac.

¶ Also an vryn white and thyn and moch in quantite w*ith* smale and longe resolutions as it is otherwhile in water that flesh is sodden in betokneth the passion that is called diabetes that {is} over mesur of making of water And this maledy cu*m*myth su*m*tym of distemp*er* of hete in the reynes. and su*m*tym be excesse of lechery. and su*m*tym of traveling. re*n*nyng or skipping vn*de* ypoc*ras* et isaac

¶ An vrin white and thyn and su*m*what yelowish or grenysh and bright it betokneth a siknes called scotomia and Vertigo. that is whan on turneth the eyes. and thi*n*keth that al the world or the howse turneth abowt hym And if it cum in hervest it betokneth a quarteyn. or a quotidian cawȝt thorow flewm vit*rie* auic*enna*. and also thorow flevm and melancoly. Ysaac and because of melancoly humers in the body vp into the hede and stopping ther *secundu*m tholomeu*m* et Egidiu*m*.

¶ Also | white vrin and thyn and a f. 4r
child betokneth coldnes of the lyu*er* Ysaac.

¶ White colo*ur* and thyn w*ith* aking and pricking and hevines aboute the spawdes *and* the shulders and the nek and namely if he haue grenis vnd*er* the cerkil betokneth a siknes called Lippotomia. i*d est*. sincopis or þe chincok. al is on. *secundu*m Walt*eriu*m et Egidiu*m*.

¶ White vrin and thyn in the day that the pacient hathe his accesse it betokneth a very quarte*i*n caused of kind malencoly but on the next day it shuld be pale or subpale or on the thurd dai or the fourth day it shuld be white or yelow and than it shal loke blakysh and thik w*ith* moch sedimen in the botom Ptolome*us*.

¶ Yf the vrin apere rubea or s*u*brubea. rufa or s*u*brufa or Citrine in the dai of the accesse it beto*k*net*h* a quartan notha. and in this wise the vrin

436 the] *cancel.* spad | **447** or[1]] *cancel.* next pale

Sedymen in þe botym. *secundum*. theo*philus*.

¶ also yf an vryn apere. Rubea. or *su*brubea. Ruffa. or *su*bruffa. or Cit*ri*ne in þe day of þe accesse it betoken*yth*. a quarteyn. notha. and i*n* þ*is* wyse þe vryn shewyth hym such in quarteyns. theo*philus*. & walte*rius*.

¶ also vryn white *and* thy*n*ne. or ȝelwe. *and* thy*n*ne. and lytel in quantyte. *and* thicke. *and* *tro*bly in þe botym. and afft*er* þ*a*t comyth an vryn moch in quantyte. þan it betokenyth warysshyng of a ffeu*er* cotidyan causyd of fflewm vit*rie*. //¶\\ and yf an vryn shewe white. *and* thy*n*ne w*ith* resoluc*io*ns lyke ffysshys scalys blacke. *and* swartte. betokenyth sykenes of þe mat*ri*ce. causyd throuh excesse of Malencoly. þe Malencoly is black. *and* swart of kynde. Egidi*us*.

¶ also. Egidi*us*. seyth þ*a*t be. iij. causis comy*n*ly þe vryn is white. somtyme because of stoppyng of hum*er*s in þe body. anamly of. Col*er*. þ*a*t þe body is euentyd to leet outt þe wyckyd hum*er*s. *and* þe excesse of hem./ the. 2. because of grete akyng. *and* pryckyng. *and* peyne in þe body. as it fallyth oftyn in oon þ*a*t hayþ þe colyca passyo./ the. 3. cause is whi the
f. 7r vryn is white. and wan. is because | of ffebylnesse of dygestyon of þe hum*er*s þe wech mow nat be defyed as þey shuld be yff dygestion wer*e* good. wer*e*for þe hum*er*s ben myxtt w*ith* þe vryn. and it is comy*n*ly i*n* þe dropsye. and this is gen*er*al signifycac*io*n of vryn þ*a*t is wat*ri* *and* wan. and also it comyn of þe lyu*er* because of such coldnesse. dygestyon is lettyd. ysaac.

¶ also an vryn white. *and* thy*n*ne w*ith* acthe. *and* peyne in þe lendys *and* þe reynes. betokenyth stoppyng of þe weyes of þe vryn because of grose fflewm // and in a ffeu*er* stoppyng of grose colr*e*. Egidi*us*.

¶ also vryn white *and* thy*n*ne þe cause is moch etyng. *and* drynkyng out of mesur*e*. and because of stoppyng of þe lyuer and betokenyth grete onhelthe. *secundu*m. theo*phi*le. & ysaac.

591 þe] *cancel.* veynes

sheweth hym souch in quarteyns. Ptolom*eus*. walter*ius* /

¶ White vrin and thin or yelow and thyn and litil in qua*n*tite and thik and trobli in the botom. and after th*at* comyth an vrin moch in qua*n*tite than it betokneth warisshing of a feuer cotidian caused of flewm vit*rie*. and if an vrin shewe white and thin w*ith* resolutions like fishes scalis blac and swart betokneth siknes of the matrice cawsed thorow excesse of melancoly. The melancoly is blac and swart of kind Egidius

¶ Egidius saith that ther be iij causes comynly the vrin is white Sumtym because of stopping of humours in the body and namly of Coler that the body is evented to let owt the wiked humours and the excesse of them / The second because of great aking and pricking ande payn in the body as it fallith often in oon that hath the colica passion The third cause is whi the vrin is white and wan is because of febelnesse of digestion of the humores the which mow not be defied as thei shuld be if digestion war good wherfor the humoures be mixte w*ith* the vrin. and it is comenly in the dropsy And this is general signification of the vrin that is watery and wan and also it co*m*myth of the liv*er* because of souch coldnesse digestion is let. Ysaac.

¶ White vrin and thyn w*ith* ache ande payn in the lendis and the reynes betokneth stopping of the wais of the vrin because of grose flewm and in a feuer stopping of grose colour Egidius.

¶ White vrin and thyn the cause therof is moche eting and drinking owt of mesure. and because of stopping of the lyver. and betokneth great helth *secundu*m Ptolom*eum* and Ysaac.

¶ And whansoeuer white vryn | is f. 4v
menely thyn w*ith* grose matter as clout*tis* in the botom than it co*m*meth of flewme vitrie Cum gleba humoris fla*m* vit*rium* hu*m*dar*e* significat no*n* putrefactu*m* *secundu*m Egidiu*m*.

467 melancoly] *ext. marg.* ¶ Melancoly

¶ and whansomeu*er* white vryn is menely thy*n*ne wyth g*ro*se mat*er* as cloutt*is* in þe botym þan it comyth of flewm vytrye. Cu*m* gleba hu*m*oris fla*m* vit*r*iu*m* hu*m*dare. sig*nificat*. no*n* putrefactu*m*. *secundu*m. Egidiu*m*.

¶ Vryn menely thy*n*ne w*ith*outt cloutt*is* betokenyth flewm acetosu*m*./ also an vryn white *and* thynne. and it ape/re\ in the begy*n*nyng of a syknes it betokenyth long syknes because of innat*ur*al hete. and of raw mat*er* // for whansomeu*er* þe mat*er* begy*n*nyth to lose. þe vryn waxyth thycke. Egidi*us*.

¶ also vryn white *and* thy*n*ne. *and* shy*n*nyng. *and* if þe shyny*n*g be somwhat toward grenesse. Malencoly. sig*nifica*t. Egidi*us*.

¶ also white *and* thy*n*ne w*ith* smal resoluc*io*ns. *and* thycke. *and* lyke long herys in þe ou*er* p*ar*ty of þe vryn. betokenyth þe artetyka passio. of Malencoly na*tur*al. Egidi*us*. & ysaac.

¶ also an vryn white *and* thy*n*ne i*n* þe Colyk. pessi*ma* e*st* Ipoc*ras*. & ysaac //¶\\ also an white *and* thy*n*ne w*ith* a ffeu*er* brenny*ng* is deth/ and yf it be w*ith*out a ffeu*er* it is coldnesse of þe
f. 7v lyu*er*. and if it be | w*ith* good signys it betokenyth a postym vnd*er* þe mydryff and yf it haue evyl signis it is deth. Egidi*us*.

¶ and yf it be white *and* thynne in þe ende of a ffeu*er* it betokenyth strenth. *and* helth of þe mylte. Egidi*us*.

¶ and if it be white. *and* thy*n*ne in a wo*m*man it betokenyth retenc*io*n of fflourys. Egidi*us*.

¶ and yf it be white. *and* thy*n*ne w*ith* smal resoluc*io*ns lyke asshys *and* somwat blackysh w*ith* scalis it betokenyth retenc*io*n of fflourys. vt di*cit* walt*er*i*us*. & Egidi*us*.

¶ also vryn white *and* thynne. bryȝt. *and* cler*e*. *and* if þe c*er*kyl. above be grene. or ledy it betokenyth þ*e* ffallyng evyl. *and* the brayn is ou*er*comyn w*ith* malencoly hum*er*s. ysaac. ¶ and yf such an vryn com in a ffeu*er* *and* lytel it betoken*yth* hasty deth. //¶\\ and yf it com in olde ffolke it betokenyth ffebylnesse of myȝtt.

644 dicit] *cancel.* of ffl

¶ Vrin menely thyn w*ith*out cloutt*is* betokneth flewm acetosu*m* Also an vrin white and thyn and it appere in the begy*nn*in*g* of the siknes it betokneth long siknesse because of innatural hete and of raw maters ffor whansoeuer the matter begin to lose the vri{n} wexeth thik. Egidi*us*.

¶ White vrin and thyn and shyni*n*g. and if the shyni*n*g be sumwhat toward grenes melancoli significat. Egidi*us*. Also white and thyn in colik pessi*ma* est Ypoc*ras* Ysaac

¶ White and thyn w*ith* smal resolutions and thik and lik longe heris in the ov*er* party of the vrin betokneth the artetica passio of malencoly n*at*ural Egid*ius*. Ysaac.

¶ White vrin and thyn w*ith* a feuer brenny*n*g is deth. and if it be w*ith*out a fever it is coldnesse of the lyver. and if it be w*ith* colde sines it betokneth an empostym vnder the mydrif. and it hath evil synys it is deth Egidius.

¶ White and thyn in the ende of a fever it betokneth strenght and helth of the mylt Egidium

¶ White and thyn in a wo*m*man it betokneth retencion of flouris Egidius

¶ White and thyn w*ith* smal resolutions as asshes and sumwhat blackish w*ith* scales it betokneth retencion of flour*is* walteri*us*. Egidi*us*.

¶ White vrin and thyn bright and clere. and if the circule above be grene or ledy it betokneth the falling evil. and the brayn is overcum with melancoly humoures. Ysaac And if souch an vrin cum in a fever. and litil. it betokneth hasti deth. and if it cum in olde folk it betokneth febelnes of myght and of kinde thorow melancoli humours Ysaac And in yong folk lacking of here sustinauns. or feuers comyng thorow melancoly. and oppressing of the sp*i*ritual membres pessi*ma* est s*ecundu*m ptolomeu*m* and the emeraud*is*

515 vrin] *emend.* urith | **552** thorow melancoly] *transp.* melancoly thorow

s*ecundu*m. Iohanem. de. sancto. amando.

¶ also an vryn white *and* thicke in þe cretyk day. anamely i*n* þe. 4. day betokenyth a postym behynde þe Erys. and affte*r* that deth. s*ecundu*m. ysaac.

¶ vryn white. *and* thyke wi*th* noo*n* ypostasys betokenyth g*ro*se and vyscouse hume*rs*. *and* pe*r*el. ysaac.

¶ vryn white *and* thick. *and* oylysh. is deth. ysaac.

¶ In all*e* these sekenes. as in þe tesyk. yd*ro*pysye. apoplexie. Epilencie. *peri*pleumo*n*ia. palsy. Colica passio. & in discenterie. yf þe vryn be red it is deth. Egidi*us*. & ysaac.

¶ also in frenesy. i*n* pluresy. in synoca. i*n* a te*r*cian yf þe vryn be white. *and* bryȝt it is deth. Egidi*us*. Walte*rius*.

Take sauge. myntte. Calamy*n*tte. p*er*sly. avence. be evyn porcyon *and* take sowre bred *and* te*mper* it {yn} wyne or stale ale. *and* pep*er*. *and* gyngre. *and* make v*er*dsauce. þ*er*of *and* vse it. anoþ*er*.

Take g*ro*myle. saxiffrage. p*er*sly. sawge and boyle hem toged*er* in stale {ale}. *and* drynke it. and vse powd*er* þ*er*of i*n* patage &c

¶ Also in frenesi in pleuresi in sinocha in a tercian Yf the vryn be white and bright it is deth Egid*ius*. Walterius.

¶ Medicina Take sauge mynt calamynt persly avence by even porcion and take soure brede and temp*er* it in wyn or stale ale and pep*er* and gynger and make verdsauce therof and vse it

¶ It*em* take gromel saxifrage p*er*sli sauge and boil them together in stale ale and drink it and vse poud*er* therof in potage etc./

f. 9r Spissi suscipiens *com*me*r*cia nulla liquoriis.
Est in iudicio glacus color emul*us* albo.
Aut min*us* offendit nature Iura coloris.
Si ffu*er*it tenuis medioc*riter* aut mediocris.
Glauka. *vel*. alba notat excessu*m* ffleu*ma*tis acris.
Glauka malencolice craseos est co*n*scia testis.
Glauka. *vel*. alba notat geranoxion plu*m*bea c*ircum*.
Alba /fre\quens multa tenuis resoluc*io* longa.
Carnea notificant si *con*ueniant diabetes.
Clarior alba c*r*isi no*n* p*re*cedente p*ro*fanat.
Continua*m* ffebrem frenesi mortale p*ro*pinq*uat*.

¶ glauke vryn. i*d est*. yelwe. it is as it //were\\ whyte shyny*ng* horn. and betokenyth as doth þe white. saff this betokenyth a lytel more hete of dygestion. for eu*er* man*er* of bryȝtnesse in vryn betokenyth drynesse. s*ecundu*m. theo*philus*.

GLAUK vrin. i*d est*. yelow it is as it war yelow colour whit shini*ng* horn and it betokneth as doth the white save this betokneth a litil mor hete of digestion ffor euery man*er* of brightnesse in vrin betokneth drynesse s*ecundu*m Ptol*omeu*m

¶ deth if he slepe nat. a long feuer. and frenesy ysac.

801 is] *cancel*. as it

780 Take] *ext. marg*. medicina | **791** emulus] *corr. by exp. and suprascr.* similis *m.r.* | **801** glauke] *ext. marg*. yelwe colo*ur*

. glauke. colour*e*.

¶ deth yf he slepe nat a long feu*er* and frensy. ysaac. Red g*ra*vel betokenyth ach. *and* a spice of the ston in þe reynes

¶ Vryn þ*a*t is white yelwesh it betokenyth syknesse in the mylte. the Cold dropsye. *and* syknes in þe reynes throuh g*ra*uel or wynde. or dru*n*kenesse. or þe ffrensy. and so to dey if it continue. or þe artica passio. or Epilencie. or tu*r*nesyke. or coldnesse of þe lyuer. *and* stoppyng þ*er*of. *and* þe mylte

¶ In olde ffolke brotylnesse of her norshyng membris or sownyng throuh sorowe and care takyng. or a ffeu*er*.
f. 9v *quart*an./ theo*philus*. | or a ffeuer cotidyan of ffleum vit*ri*e. or retenc*i*on of wo*m*me*n*s ffloury*s*. //¶\\ and in men þe Emrawdys. and such*e* oþ*er* maledyes of þe ars. s*ecundu*m. Gilb*ertum*. & Gordianu*m*. auic*enna*.

¶ also yelwe vryn menely thycke. tokenyth malencoly bothe in men. and wo*m*me*n*. Walt*erius*. aueroy.

¶ also an vryn þ*a*t is more thycke þan thy*n*ne of yelwe colour betokenyth an egr*e* fflewm. theo*philus*.

¶ also vryn of glauke colour*e* tokenyth mor*e* indigestioun //. and malencoli·\\ þan doth white colo*ur*./ and yf it be thy*n*ne substaunce w*ith* clowtt*is* in þe botym. *and* wyndy. w*ith*out feu*er* it is of flewm vit*rie*. *and* grete peyne. *and* p*er*ell. Gordyan*us*.

¶ also yelwe vryn w*ith* a thy*n*ne substau*n*ce. sig*nificat*. salute*m*. Egidi*us*.

¶ þ*er* be. v. man*er* of flewmys. fflewma. naturalis. fflewma. dulce. fflewma. salsu*m*. fflewma acetosu*m*. fflewma. vitreu*m*. ysaac.

Take. ffenel rot*is*. the Iuse of tansy. h*er*be benet. ysope. my*n*tte. sawge. Centory. p*er*sly. sp*a*rag*us*. gingr*e*. lycoriys. *and* ho/n\y. all*e* this soden in wyn. *and* drynke it.

Soluit & a mortis laqueis emancipat egru*m*.
In ffebre qua*m* replicat tipic*usque* int*er*polat error.

850 Take] *ext. marg.* medicina | **855** Soluit] *ext. marg.* Lacteus

855 laqueis] Read as *lacteus*

¶ White yelowish vrin betokneth siknesse in the mylt the colde dropsy and siknesse in the reynes. thorow gravel or winde or drunkenes or the frenesy. and so to dey if it co*n*tynow. or the artica passio. or Epilencie or tu*r*nesik or coldnes of the lyver and stopping therof and of the mylt.

¶ In old folkes brotilnes of her norishing membres or sowning thorow sorow or care taking or a feuer quarte*i*n Ptolomeus. or a feuer quotidian of flewme vit*r*ie. or Retencion of womans floures. and in men the emeraud*is* and such other maladis of the arse s*ecundu*m Gilbertu*m* Gordianu*m* et Auicen*na*.

¶ Yelow vrin menely thik betokneth melancoly both in men and wo*m*men Walteri*us* Aueroys

¶ Vrin more thik than thyn of yelow colour betokneth an eg*re* fleume Ptolome*us*

¶ Glauc vrin if it be of thyn substance w*ith* clout*is* in the bottom and windy w*ith*out feu*er* it is of flewm vit*r*ie and great payn and perel Gordian*us*

¶ Yelow vrin w*ith* a thyn substance significat salutem Egidius

¶ fflegma. Naturale. Dulce. Salsum. Acetosum. Vitrie.

¶ Take fenel rotis. the Ius of tansey h*er*be benet isop mynt sauge Centory p*er*sly sp*a*rag*us* ginger Licoris and hony al soden in wyn and drink it.

700 an] *cancel.* og

708 fflegma] *bot. marg.* ¶ τελόσ

lacte/a\ subtenuis dicat quod causa sit eius.
frigida p*re*ssura longi ffactura laboris.
lactea subtenuis febre declinante salute*m*.
Impet*rat* et corp*us* elevat vitamq*ue* reformat.
lactea s*u*btenuis cu*m* largo fusa liquoris.
ffine mali venie*n*s de frenesce*n*te calore.
lactea s*u*btenuis in acute caumate febris.
l/a\ctis in /ingressu\ signis adiu*n*cta sinistris.
f. 10r dampnat. & accusat paciente*m* *crimin*e mortis.
ffallit*ur* vrine sentencia si tibi certo.
Ordine concurrant que su*n*t vitalia signa.
Mens. Sapor. affect*us* bona. respiraci*o* vi*r*tus.

. Milky. colo*ur*.
¶ deth yf he slepe nat. a ffrenesy.

¶ vryn of milky colo*ur* it is whitt*er* þan is alb*us* and is causyd throuh flewmatyk hum*er*s. and it be thy*n*ne a feu*er* it is deth. anamely if þ*er* com wyckyd signis þ*er*wyth as /no\ reste. spuyng. vnky*n*d slepe. walwyng. shrot breth. mevyng his handys. pyckyng þe walle. or hys nosethyrlys. *and* such*e* oþ*er* moo. Walt*erius*.

¶ also vryn lacte*us* *and* lytel betoken*yth* deth. Gilb*ertus* ¶ and thouh it be lytel. or the*n*ne w*ith* good signis. it betokenyth warysshyng. *and* lyff. Egidi*us*.

¶ also vryn lacte*us* thy*n*ne. *and* moch in qua*n*tyte in þe ende of a feu*er* betokenyth þe tysyk. Egidi*us*. //¶\\ and also it betokenyth þe dropsye w*ith* all oþ*er* sykenessis aforeseyd in alba. and glauka. Walt*erius*. ysaac.

¶ also this vryn thycke ou*er* all betokenyth fleu*m* natural. s*ecundu*m. Ioh*an*em de s*a*ncto am*a*ndo. & Gordian*us*. //¶\\ and yf it be thy*n*ne ou*er* all male*n*coli. sig*nifica*t. s*ecundu*m. Io*hanem*. de. s*ancto*. a*mando*.

¶ and /it\ be menly thy*n*ne it betokenyth flewm acetosu*m* ¶ yf it be passyng thy*n*ne *and* moch in qua*n*tyte weth*er* com in þe begy*n*nyn*g* or þe endyng it betokenyth warysshyng. //*and* helthe. Egidi*us*.\\

f. 10v ¶ Vryn lacte*us*. and menely thycke

864 /ingressu\] *cancel.* nigre

857 lacte/a\] *ins.* lacte/a\ *m.r.* | **861** liquoris] *corr. by exp. and suprascr.* liquor/e\ *m.r.* | **862** frenescente] *corr. by exp. and suprascr.* fervesce*n*te *m.r.* | **864** /ingressu\] *suprascr. m.r.* | **865** crimine] *corr. by exp. and suprascr.* crimine *m.r.*

f. 6r MYLKYE vrin it is whiter than is albus and is caused thorow fleumatik humoures and it be thyn a fev*er* it is dethe and namly if ther cu*m* wicked signes therw*ith* as no rest. spuyng. vnkind slepe. waluyng shorte breth meving his hand*is*. picking the wal. or his nosethirls and souch other moo Walteri*us*

¶ Mylky vrin ande litil betokneth dethe Gilbertus And though it be litil or thyn w*ith* good signes it betokneth warishing of Lif Egidius.

¶ Milky vrin and thyn and moch in quantite in the ende of /a\ feu*er* betokneth the ptisik Egidius. Also it betokneth the dropsy w*ith* al other siknes aforsaid in alba et glauca Walteri*us* Ysaac

¶ Also this vrin thik ov*er* al betokneth flewm natural s*ecundu*m Io*hanem* d*e* s*ancto* a*mando*. et Gordianu*m* And if it be thyn over al melancoly sig*nifica*t s*ecundu*m Io*hannes* d*e* s*ancto* a*mando*.

And it be meneli thyn it betokneth flewm acetosu*m* yf it be passing thyn and moch in qua*n*tite whether it cum in the begi*n*ni*n*g or in thending it betokneth warisshing and helth Egidius

¶ Milky vrin and me{n}ely thik w*ith* clout*is* in the botom betokneth a feuer quotidian of flewm vitrie and corrupt Gilbert*us*

¶ Milky vrin and karapos thik litil and trobly w*ith* long resolutions or rownd betokneth loseny*n*g of the beli Egidius. And it be w*ith* resolutions in

746 menely] *emend.* metely

w*ith* clouttis *in* þe botym betokenyth a ffeu*er* Cotidian of fflewm vit*r*ie *and* corrupt. //Gil*bertus*.\\

¶ also vryn lacte*us* or karapos thicke lytel *and* t*ro*bly wyth long resoluc*io*ns or rownd betokenyth loseny*ng* in the bely. Egidi*us*. ¶ and it be w*ith* resoluc*io*ns in the botym as it wer*e* asshys. it betoken*yth* diariam þ*at* is þ*e* fflyx. Walt*erius*.

¶ also vryn lacte*us*. or livid*us*. derke. *and* thicke in wo*m*men it betokenyth retencion of flourys. Gilb*ertus*.

¶ also vryn white lyke sp*er*me betokenyth a postym þ*at* is bred of fflwem vit*r*ie. *and* apoplexia. aueroiȝ. 4º. *capitu*lo./

¶ and if it be white. *and* lytel and lyke sp*er*me it betokenyth þe palsye. Ras*us*. 10. a*ni*maliu*m*.

¶ also vryn lyke sp*er*me betokenyth grete cold and dyssoluyng of sykenesse in þe guttys. *con*stantin*us*. 7º. pantegni.

¶ also vryn lacteus somtyme betokenyth. þ*at* a. ma*n* is broste w*it*h*y*nne. and his bowell*is* fallyn down into his codde. auycen*na*.

a medicyn þ*er*for.

Take rosen. wax. ffrankensence. mastyk. swy*n*nys grece oyle olyve. and medle all toged*er*. þan take powd*er* of comyn. *and* of lynsed of anys sed. of ffynkell sed *and* medyl all toged*er*. and make a plast*er* on leder*e*. *and* ley it on the dyssese. saff ley a ly*n*nen cloth betwyn þe plast*er*. *and* the sore

//¶\\ also take matfelo*u*n. co*n*ffery and dayssey. *and* osm*u*nd. and stampe all toged*er*. *and* yeve hym to drynke w*ith* stale ale erly on morwe *and* late at eue*n* //¶\\ and lett hym absteyn hy*m* from gowt*us* met*is* *and* dry*n*k*is*. as onyo*u*ns. lek*is*. garlek. sourebred nor t*ra*uel. nor ete no potage nor sewys nor no swllyng met*is*. *and* this shall hele hym &c.

f. 11r ¶ also þe sed of white popy. and make oyle. or an oy*n*ment of henbane. *and* anoy*n*te þe templys þ*er*w*ith*.

916 wommen] *ext. marg.* mulier | **923** sperme] *ext. marg.* sperme | **934** Take] *ext. marg.* medic/i\na

the botom as it war ashis it betokneth diarion that is the flux Walteri*us*

¶ Vrin lactei or liuide derke and thik in women it tokneth retention of flouris Gilbert*us*

¶ Vrin whit like sp*er*me toknethe a postym that is brede of {flewm} vitrie and appoplexia. Au*eroes* 4º c*apitu*lo

¶ Yf it be white and litil like sperme it tokneth the palsey Ras*us* Xº Ani*ma*liu*m*.

¶ Vrin like sp*er*me tokneth great cold and dissoluy*ng* of siknesse in the guttis Co*n*stantin*us* 7 pantegni

¶ Also vrin lacte*us* su*m*tym tokneth that a man is brust w*ith*in and his bowellis falt downe into his cod. Auic*enna*

¶ MEDICINA þ*er*for.

Take rosen wax francincense mastik swines grese oil olif and medil al together Than take poud*er* of comyn and of linsed and of anissede of fenkel sede and medil al together *and* make a plaster of lether and lei it on the disease save ley a lynen cloth betwen the plaster and the sor*e*

¶ Also take mat felon co*n*fery and daysey and osmu*n*d and stamp al together and gef hym to drink w*ith* stale ale erli on the morow and late at evyn and let hym absteyn from gowt*is* met*is* and drinkes as onyons Lekis garleke soure brede nor travale nor ete no potage nor sewes nor no swelling metis. and this shal hele hym

¶ Also the sede of white popi and make oyl. or an oyntment of henban and annoynt the temples therwithe.

be moste toward white w*ith* a contynual spume it betoken*yth* peripleumon*i*a. s*ecundu*m. Iohan*em*. de. s*ancto*. amand*o*.

¶ also vryn. karapos fatt above in the begy*n*nyng of a ffeu*er* betokenyth moch wynde. and yf it com afft*er* þ*at* moch vryn. *and* thy*n*ne it betoken*yth*. a. *con*tin*u*al ffeu*er*./ theo*philus*.

Take and avente the in þe legg*is*. and vse croppys of sawge w*ith* tr*i*acle dru*n*kyn þ*er*. *and* bugle.

Pallida cu*m* pingui. *ve*l. subcitr*i*na liquore.
ffleumatice monstr*at* pe*r*iodica ffrigora ffebris.
Palida cu*m* tenui col*eram* declarat adustam.
Pallida subtenuis ex acre flewmate febr*em*.
Pallida cui spissu*m* mediocr*i*ter associat*ur*.
f. 12v ffleumatice craseos interp*res* fida p*ro*bat*ur*.
Si male disposito p*re*cedat corp*ore* glauka.
Lactea. *vel*. karapos. & pallida p*ost* videat*ur*.
Signo palloris vires natura resumit.
Et redit ad p*ropriu*m vis digestiua tenore*m*.
In febre *con*tinua lenta subpallida clara.
Pond*us* apostaseos in dext*ra* pa*r*te futur*um*.
Indicat affecte *con*stante vigente vigore.
Si ffluor absentet uentris *aut* viscera te*m*ptet.
Pallida spumosa pinguis liuens cin*er*osa.
Paucula sit pestis ptisice no*n* *con*sona test*is*.
Si fluor accedit.mors /intrat\ vita recedit.
Crudor. & eufraxis ffl*u*x*us* *con*su*m*pc*i*o pauca.
Indicat vrina*m* rac*i*o *contr*aria multam.

¶ Now for to knowe pale colour. it is as it wer*e* the galle of a neete wer*e* meyntt w*ith* a good qua*n*tite of wat*er*. than þe colo*ur* þ*at* comyth of bothe is pale or palysh. theo*philus*. & Egidi*us*. walt*eriu*s. aueroiȝ.

. Pallidus.

¶ A bre*n*nyg vnd*er* þe lyu*er*. a febyl hed. a bad stomak. wastyng of the lu*ngis*.

. Subpallidus.

¶ A postym in þe ryȝt syde. *and* the tysyk. hard to make water.

1069 tenui] *cancel.* tenuis | **1083** /intrat\] *cancel.* venit

1064 Take] *ext. marg.* medicina | **1070** acre] *corr. by suprasc.* acr/i\ *m.r.* | **1072** interpres] *corr. by exp. and suprascr.* interpres *m.r.* | **1078** apostaseos] *ins. by suprascr. id est* collecti apostematis *m.r.* | parte] *ins. by suprascr. id est* ypocondrie *m.r.* | **1079** vigente vigore] *transp.* vigore vigente *m.r.* | **1082** consona] *corr. by exp. and suprascr.* /ab\sona *m.r.* | **1083** /intrat\] *suprascr. m.r.*

1084 eufraxis] Read as a form of euphrasia

winde and if ther cu*m* after þ*at* moch vrin and thyn it tokneth a contrary feuer Ptolom*eus*.

¶ Take and avent the in the leggis and vse croppis of sage with triacle dronken and bugle

Pale
NOW for to know. PALE colour it is as it war the gal of a nett war meynt w*ith* a good quantite of water than the color that co*m*myth of both is pale or yelowish Ptolomeus. Egidius. Walterius Auerois.

¶ bre*n*ny*n*g vnder the liuer. a feble hed. a bad stomoc. wasting of lu*ngis*.

¶ a postym in thright side the tisik. hard to make water./

¶ And coler be meynt with flewme than it is of pale colore ffor if ther ware no colour ell*is* the vryn war but alba or glauca or Lactea or karapos and therfor if pale cu*m* after these iiij it tokneth that kind begy*n*neth to haue the maistery and worketh and scaterith wicked humours first colera

887 pale] *top. marg.* pale

f. 13r ¶ and col*er* be mey*n*gtt w*ith* fleume þan it is of pale colo*ur*. Egidi*us*. //¶\\ for yf þ*er* were no col*er*. ellis þe vryn wer*e* but. alba. or glauca. or lactea. or karapos. //¶\\ and þ*er*for yf pale cu*m* aft*er* these. iiij. it betokenyth þ*at* kynde begy*n*nyth to haue þe mayst*ri*. and worchyth. *and* skateryth wyckyd hum*er*s fyrst Col*er* for he is moste sotyl to be dysp*ar*blyd. Galt*erius*.

//. a tysyk or an Etyk *and* aft*er* that com. diaria. þ*at* is a fflux it is deth. Gil*bertus*.\\

¶ Vryn pale or s*ub*pale w*ith*. a feu*er*. betokenyth rewm and compacc*ion*. þ*at* is warryng or lu*m*pyng of mat*er*. *and* if þ*er* com a tysyk þ*er*afft*er* it betoken*yth* deth. Galt*erius*.

¶ also vnd*er*stond þ*is* for a rewle they þ*at* han þe tesyk or an Etyk comy*n*ly aȝens her*e* deth. *and* a fflux. and because of þe feu*er*. þe kyndly hete. *and* þe spi*ri*t*is*. and þe myȝtt*is* of þe body ben so wastyd. *and* dyst*ro*yd. and þe kyndly moystnesse /is\ co*n*su*m*pte. //¶\\ and in þe fflux is ȝytt mor*e* p*er*dyc*ion* *and* more *con*su*m*pc*ion* of þe spirit*is*. and of kyndly hete. *and* of moystnesse and þ*er* throwh bothe kynde is moch wastyd. ypocras.

¶ also vryn pale or s*ub*pale w*ith* a thy*n*ne s*ub*stau*n*ce it betokenyth a feu*er* of sowr*e* fflewm. *and*. a postym to com vnd*er* þe riȝtte syde. //*and* col*er* aduste.\\ *and* long syknes. auicen*na*.

¶ also vryn pale or s*ub*pale. moch*e* *and* thy*n*ne w*ith* att*ur* as gleba in þe botym betokenyth þe st*r*anguryon anamely yf it be white. auic*enna*. & Galt*erius*. ¶ and yf it be lytel þe fflux of þe wo*m*be. auic*enna*.

//¶\\ also vryn pale or s*ub*pale com aft*er* cit*ri*ne. and þan karapos. salutem. sig*nifica*t. ypoc*ras*. Egidi*us*.

¶ vryn pale *and* thy*n*ne somwhat t*ur*nyn*g* to g*re*nesse betokenyth grete adustio*un* of malencoly. Egidi*us*.

¶ vryn pale *and* thy*n*ne somwhat t*ur*nyn*g* to whitnesse betokenyth adustio*un* of flewm. Egidi*us*. //¶\\ and

for that is most sotellest to be dispersed Galterius

¶ And after that a ptisik and an etik and after that cu*m* diaria. that is a flux it is deth Gilbertus

¶ Vryn pale or subpale w*ith* a fever tokneth rewme and co*m*paction that is warring or lumping of matter and if ther cu*m* a tisik after it tokneth deth Galterius

¶ Also vnderstond this for a reule ¶ That thei that haue the tisik and an etik comenly ayenst ther deth a flux and because of the feuer a kindly hete and the sprit*is* and the myght*is* of the bodi be so wasted and destroied and the kindli moistnes is | consumpte. f. 7v
and in the flux ys it more perdicion and more co*n*su*m*ption of the sprigtys. and of kindly hete. and of moystnes and ther thorow both kindly hete and of moistnes and ther thorow both kind is moch lost and wasted. Ypoc*ras*

¶ Pale vrin or subpale w*ith* a thyn substanc*e* it tokneth a feuer of soure flewm and a postom to cu*m* vnd*er* the right side and coler aduste and long siknesse Auic*enna*

¶ Pale vrin or subpale moch and thin as att*er* as gleba in the botom betokneth the strangurion and namely if it be white Auic*enna* Galteri*us* And if it be litil the flux of the wombe Auic*enna*

¶ Pale vrin or subpale cu*m* after citrine and than karapos salute*m* significat Ypoc*ras* Egidius

¶ Pale and thyn su*m*what turnyng to grenenysh tokneth great adustion of melancoly Egidius

¶ Pale and su*m*what thyn su*m*what turny*ng* to whitnesse tokneth adustion of fleume Egid*ius* and hit be toward glauk color melancoly naturale*m* sig*nifica*t Egid*ius*

¶ Pale and menely thik sig*nifica*t admixtione flegmat*is* ¶ Pale and thyn and su*m*what shadowed above tokneth begy*n*nyng of digestio*un* Eg*idius* Gal*ienus*

1131 and] *rep.* and

1116 rewle] *ext. marg.* Re*wle*

947 hit] *cancel.* to be toward

it be toward liuid*us*. col*er*ram sig*nificat* Egidius //¶\\ and it be toward clauke colo*ur*. malencolica*m* naturale*m* sig*nifica*t. Egidi*us*.

f. 13v ¶ also vryn pale and menely thycke sig*nifica*t admixtio*ne*ȝ. fleu*matis*. //¶\\ also vryn pale *and* thy*n*ne. *and* somwhatt shadwyd. above betokenyth begy*n*nyng of dygestio*un*. Egidi*us*. & Galien*us*.

¶ also vryn pale. or s*u*bpale w*ith* a thy*n*ne s*u*bsta*u*nce w*ith* soppys *and* gobett*is* in þe botym. *and* brokyn. abrode betokenyth grete torcio*un*. *and* ventosyte in þe bely. and it comyth of flewm vytrie. Galt*er*i*us*. Gilb*er*t*us*. Gordian*us*. li*bro*. p*ri*mo. ca*pitul*o. de coti*di*ana notha

¶ also vryn s*u*bpale thy*n*ne. *and* clere w*ith* a *con*ti*nual* feu*er* w*ith* oþ*er* good signys. as good my*n*de. appetite. strength. v*er*tu. not esy fettyng of wynde betokenyth. a postym to com vnd*er* þe ryȝt syde. and long sykenesse. *and* it be *contra*ry it is deth. Egidi*us*.

¶ Vryn pale and ffatty. *and* spumose. above. and lytell in qua*n*tyte betoken*yth* þe flux. þe tesyk. *and* deth. anamely yf it be an asshy. or. a lividi colo*ur*. Egidi*us*. & Galien*us*.

¶ vryn pale w*ith* depnes of colo*ur*. or liȝtnes of colo*ur*. and litel in qua*n*tite w*ith* many resoluc*i*ons as asshis. *and* such oth*er*. and be sep*ar*att in þe ou*er* regio*un*. ffluxu*m*. ve*n*tris sig*nifica*t. Galien*us*.

¶ vryn pale and oylysh. *and* litel in qua*n*tite. *and* liȝtt. above w*ith* resoluc*i*ons as squames. or ffurphurijs. p*ri*maȝ. speci*e*ȝ ethice sig*nifica*t.

//¶\\ and yf it be ffatte w*ith* þe *con*te*n*tis aforseyd ou*er* all þe vryn it betokenyth the. secu*n*d spice of þe Etyk ¶ and it haue all*e* þe signis afor*e*seyd. and liȝtt above w*ith* resoluc*i*ons Crynoides it betokenyth. þe. 3. spice of þe Etyk. vt di*cit* Galien*us* i*n* *con*te*n*t*is*.

¶ vryn pale passyng thy*n*ne. or passyng thicke w*ith* a gr*o*se spume. *and* a*m*pullosa. betokenyth vyscouse.

1175 deth] *ext. marg.* deth | **1179** deth] *ext. marg.* deth | **1194** Etyk] ext. marg. þe Etyk

¶ Pale or subpale w*ith* a thyn substance w*ith* soppis and gobettis in the bottom and broken abrode tokneth great torsion and ventosite in the bely and it cu*m*meth of flewm vitrie Galteri*us* Gilbert*us* Gordianus li*bro* p*ri*mo ca*pitul*o de coti*di*ana notha

¶ Subpale. thyn. and clere w*ith* a contrary feuer w*ith* other good signes. as good mynd. appetit. strenght. not ease fetting of breth betokneth a postym to cum vnd*er* the right side and long siknes. and it be contrary it is deth Egidius

¶ Pale ande fatti. and spumouse above and litil in qua*n*tite tokneth the flux the tisik and dethe and namely if it be an asshe or a lividi color Egid*ius* Gale*n*

¶ Pale w*ith* depnesse of colour or litnesse of colour and litil in qua*n*tite w*ith* many resolutions as asshis and such other and be sep*ar*at in the over region fluxu*m* ventris sig*nifica*t Galen.

¶ Pale oylish and litil in quantite and light above w*ith* resolutions as squa*m*mes or furfurijs prima*m* spec*ie*m ethice sig*nifica*t

¶ And if it be fat w*ith* the contentis aforsayd over al the vrin it tokneth the second spice of the Etik. And it haue al the synes aforesaid and light above w*ith* resolutions Crinoides it tokneth the thirde spice of the etik vt dicit galenus in conte*n*t*is*

¶ Pale passing thyn or passing thik with a grose spume and ampullosa tokneth viscouse and crude and sik humours Gilbert*us* Egidius

¶ Pale fat. and trobly and thyn and low of colour and red gravel tokneth great peyn in the reynes w*ith* sleping of the fete And if the gravel be white it is of the bladder. and if it be moch | f. 8r
thyn or moch thik or of colour hy or low red or white w*ith* heris in the botom it tokneth great peyn and stopping and drynes in that placis Galteri*us*

¶ Subpale. or glauc. or karapos. w*ith*

1002 peyn] *cancel.* in the bott

and crude. *and* syke hum*er*s. Galt*eriu*s. & Egidi*us*.

¶ vryn pale ffatt *and* trobly. *and* the*n*ne. *and* louh of colo*ur*. *and* red gravel betokenyth grete peyne in þe reynes w*ith* slepyng of þe ffett. and yf f. 14r þe gr*a*uel be white it is of þe bladder | and yf it be moch thy*n*ne or moch thicke or of colour*e* hiȝe or lowh red or white w*ith* herys in þe botom it betokenyth grete peyne *and* stoppyng. *and* drynes i*n* þe plac*is*. s*ecundu*m. //Galt*erium*.\\

¶ also vryn subpale. or glauke. or karapos w*ith* asshis resydent in þe botom betokenyth grete peyne in þe brest w*ith* moch cold mat*er* of evyl *com*plexio*u*n. Galt*eriu*s.

¶ also pale vryn thy*n*ne *and* lyȝtt. & tru*m*bosa i*m* ffu*n*do albi coloris st*ra*nguriam. sig*nifica*t. Galt*eriu*s.

¶ also yf vryn pale or s*u*bpale be thyck of substau*n*ce in þe myddys it betokenyth streytnes at þe brest and glett at þe herte. theo*philus*. & ypoc*ra*s.

Take lyu*er*wort. spyg*er*nel. hertystu*n*g. turmentyll. all lych moch *and* boylyd in good ale to þe. 3. p*ar*t. dry*n*k it.

Take þe Croppys of hor*e*hound. *and* the rotys of mylffoyle. *and* bray hem in a mort*er* *and* put þ*er*to warm ale *and* streyne it throuh a cloth. and ȝeue hym to drynke at. 3. tymes ffastyng. anoþ*er*.

¶ R*ecipe*. mirabolan Iudicu*m*. aloen epatyk. sene. gete. tu*n*cressed. bromsed. *and* vse þis. //¶\\ and yf þe vryn be w*i*th a thy*n*ne s*u*bstau*n*ce i*n* þe mydel it betokenyth ffeyntness of all þe body. auic*enna*.

Take a quart of þi own pysse. *and* sethe it and put þ*er*to co*m*myn a ob*ulus* *and* let hi*m* stond þ*er* ou*er* *and* þan let hi*m* be had to bedd *and* wrappyd close in shet*is*. &c.

Est multis tenuis cit*r*ina referta figuris.
fflewmaticu*m* iuuene*m*. *v*el. que*m* nig*er* afficit humor.

asshis residence in the botom tokneth great payn in the brest w*ith* moch cold matter of evil complexion Galteri*us*

¶ Pale vrin thyn and light et tenebrosa in fundo albi coloris stranguriam sig*nifica*t Galteri*us*

¶ Pale or subpale being thik of substanc*e* in the myddes it tokneth streightnes at the brest and glet at the hart theophilus Ypoc*ras*

¶ Medicina Take liuerwort pymp*er*nel hartistong turmentyl al alich moch *and* boil it in good ale to the thred p*ar*te and so drink it

¶ Take the croppis of horhound and the rotis of mylfoil and bray hem in a morter and put therto warme ale and streyn it thorow a cloth and yeve hym to drink at iij tymes fasting

¶ Take mirabolan iudicu*m* aloen epatik cene gete tu*n*cressede bromesede and vse this. and if the vryn be w*ith* a thyn substance in the medel it tokneth feitnesse of al the body Auic*enna*

¶ Take a quarte of thy own vryn and sethe it. and put therto comyn an ob*olus* and let hym stond theron and than let hym be had to bed and wrapped close in shetis.

1206 gravel] ext. marg. þe ston | **1228** Take] *ext. marg.* medicina | **1232** Take] int. marg. oþ*er* | **1241** vryn] *ext. marg.* vryn | **1244** Take] *ext. marg.* A medicyn þerffor

na*tur*al. *secundum* Iohanem de *sancto* amando

¶ also vryn cit*r*ine. *and* almost lyke su{b}rubea. *and* sotyl and yardy. *and* cloudy. sig*nificat*. mel*ancolia*ȝ. Galt*erius*. //¶\\ neu*er*þelesse þe day aft*er* the accesse it is hott*er* þan þe day þ*at* it is on. in þe wech day it is glauke. or pale. *and* betoken*yth* syknes of þe splen. Egidi*us*.

¶ also vryn cit*r*ine *and* most thy*n*ne above w*ith* this *con*te*n*te ampull*e* *and* *gr*anys vnd*er* þe c*er*kyl betokenyth grete peyne in the breste. and the tysyk. Egidi*us*.

¶ vryn derke *and* sotyl betokenyth adustyon. *and* stoppy*n*g. *and* drying of þe body *and* of þe splen. Egidi*us*.

¶ also a vryn cit*r*ine thy*n*ne *and* moch in quantyte betoken*yth* drynes. *and* leennesse of þe body. and *con*stipat in þe bely. *and* drynesse of þe lyu*er*. w*ith* peyne vnd*er* þe ryȝtt syde. *and* fflewm rysyng up to þe throte w*ith* an hote *and* a drye ffume. auic*enna*.

¶ also vryn cit*r*ine almost lyke subrubea w*ith* yardys w*ith* þe c*er*kyl *tur*ny*n*g into *gr*ene col*our*. it betokenyth adustyon of the lyu*er*. Walt*erius*. Egidi*us*.

¶ also vryn cit*r*ine ffatty. *and* oyly. w*ith* spume as greynys. betokenyth þe tesyk. *and* þe couh. ysaac. ypoc*ras*. walt*erius*.

¶ also vryn cit*r*ine or subcit*r*ine passyng. and yardy in þe myddys. it is a postym þ*at* is callyd pluresys. //¶\\ *and* it be moch in qua*n*tyte it is sykenes of þe lyu*er*. //¶\\ *and* it be lytell it is sykenes in breste. //¶\\ and

f. 16r in chyldryn the lesse | Emit*r*iceu*m*. *secundum*. Ioh*an*em de. S*ancto* amando.

Take Scabyose. h*er*be benet. sauge. hore*h*ound. Elenaca*m*pana ysope. ffigg*is*. lycorys. and boyle hem in galon of wat*er* to a potel. and vse to drynke it oftyn. ano*þer*.

Take powd*er* of polipody and aloe Epatyk *and* medyl these toged*er* w*ith* sugr*e* and vse it in potage.

1386 Take] *ext. marg.* medicina

and co*n*stipat in the bely and drynesse of the lyuer w*ith* payn vnder the right side. and flewm rising vp to the throte and w*ith* an hote and a dry fume auic*enna*.

¶ Citrin almost like subrubea w*ith* yard*is* w*ith* the circul turnyng into grene colour it tokneth adustion of the lyver Walter*ius*. Egid*ius*.

¶ Citrine fatty and oyly w*ith* spume as greynes tokneth the tisik and the cowghg Ysa*ac*. Ypoc*ras*. Wal*terius*.

¶ Citrin or subcitrin passing and yardi in | the myddis is a postym that is f. 9r
called Pleuresis And it be moch in qua*n*tite it is siknesse of the lyver and it be litil it is siknesse in the brest and in children the {l}esse emen*tricium* *secundum* Io*hanem* d*e* *sancto* a*mando*

¶ Medicina ¶ Take scabious herbe benet saug horhound enula campana isop figg*is* licor*is* and boil hem in a galon of water to a potel and vse to drink it often

¶ It*em* Take pou*de*r of polipody and aloe Epatik, and medle these together w*ith* sug*re* and vse it in potage.

¶ vj maner of colers Colera Naturalis Nigra Citrina Viridis prassina Eruginosa. galen.

1122 the[2]] *cancel.* R | **1134** in] *rep.* in | **1138** lesse] *emend.* sesse þ*er* be. v. man*er* of col*er*is. col*er*a natural*is*. col*er*a citrina. col*er*a viridis. col*er*a nigra. col*er*a viridis. col*er*a prassina. col*er*a Eruginosa. Galyen.

In ruffu*m* vergens pure color emul*us* auri.
Equalis medi*us* pur*us* cui se liquor vnit.
In puero iuuene sene flewmatico muliere.
Ruffa manens tenuis notat. *hoc.* incom*m*oda febris.
Co*n*tinua*m* t*r*iceu*m* duplice*m sed* temp*or*e longo.
Epatis offensa*m*. *v*el. ffebre*m* quat*r*iduana*m*.
P*r*incipio cause du*m* su*n*t nova se*min*a morbi.
Rufa paru*m* tenuis cui*us* su*m*ma*m* cui*us* regione*m*.
Nubes rara tenet. motu gen*er*ata caloris.
De salso tipitycam succe*n*dit fflewmate febre*m*.
S*ed* t*r*iceu*m* morbo iam p*r*ocedente figurat.
Spissa par*um* ia*m* no*n* t*r*iceu*m* magis indusiosa*m*.
In exsalso. *v*el. dulci fflewmate ffebre*m*.
fflewmat*is* ex salsi mordax exuberat humor.
f. 16v Et sine ffebre fuerit enormes excitat act*us*.
Extremans pu*n*gens feruoris acumine p*ar*tes.
Si subruffa par*um* tenuis no*n* nubila fiat.
Et talem s*er*uet *con*stanti tempora forma*m*.
ydropico talis p*or*tenditur excisialis.
//¶\\ Rufa par*um* pinguis retinens u*m*b*r*acula nub*is*.
Indicat accendi febre*m* de flewmati dulce.
Infra s*u*bcistit calor uel s*u*bstancia constet.
fflewmatis excess*us* dulc*is*. sine febre notat*ur*.
Ruffa par*um* tenuis. *v*el. pinguis liuida constans.
Membra quib*us* fiunt spiramina flewmate dulce.
Vel salso mo*n*strat certa rac*i*one grauari.
In muliere magis p*or*tendit probra monete.
//¶\\ Si color e*st* Ruffus pinguis substancia febre*m*.
Signat continua*m* de fleumate vasa tene*n*te.
Si sit causa recens. & su*m*mu*m* liuor obu*m*brat.
Aut minor innuit*ur*. aut pluresis i*n*sinuat*ur*.
Si vet*us* alchites mag*is* aut empima vocat*ur*.

1413 Et] *cancel.* si

1398 auri] *ext. marg.* Gold colo*ur* | **1401** hoc] *corr. by exp.* hec *m.r.* | **1403** sed] *corr. by exp.* si *m.r.* | **1404** offensam] *corr. by exp. and suprascr.* effusam *m.r.* | **1406** summam cuius] *transp.* cui*us* summam *m.r.* | **1408** De] *corr. by exp. and suprascr.* In *m.r.* | **1410** indusiosam] *ins. by suprascr. id est* fiver cotidiana*m* | **1411** In] *corr. by exp. and suprascr.* indicat *m.r.* | **1412** ex] *corr. by exp. and suprascr.* et *m.r.* | **1413** fuerit] *corr. by exp.* //humor fure*ns*\\ *m.r.* | **1415** nubila] *corr. by exp.* //nebula\\ *m.r.* | **1420** calor uel] *corr. by exp. and suprascr.* c/o\lor et *m.r.* | **1423** spiramina] *corr. by exp. and suprascr.* spirantia *m.r.* | dulce] *corr. by exp. and suprascr.* dulc/i\ *m.r.* | **1429** innuitur] *corr. by exp. and suprascr.* mutatur *m.r.*

1403 triceum duplicem] *Duplex* could also be taken alongside *triceum* to denote a six-day period | **1417** excisialis] Read as *excitialis*, a variant spelling of *exitialis*

Si spumosa mag*is* fiat cin*er*isq*ue* coloris.
Debile rewm/a\tica me*m*br*um* t*ur*bante qurela.
Disponi pot*er*it pinguis pot*er*it rufi q*ue* coloris.
Si spumosa mag*is* fiat cin*er*isq*ue* coloris.
Em/u\la distincte liue*ns* s*u*brufa remissa.
Ad loca pulmo*n*is lat*er*is morb*us* peregr*in*at.
Pynguis rufa par*um* liue*ns* oleagena crinis.
Obsita fit febris Etice legata fidelis.

f. 17r ¶ Rufe *and* subruffe ffolwyn by ord*er* afft*er* Cit*r*ine. and is of mene colo*ur* betwyn Cit*r*ine *and* red. Ioh*an*em de sancto amando.

. Ruffus.
¶ The Emraudys. d*r*opsy. passyng of fflouris. ffeyntnes of wat*er* betokenyth streytnes at þe brest and a ffeu*er*.
. Subruffus.
¶ A ffeu*er*. an e*m*postem vnd*er* þe rybbis. *and* þe artetica passio *and* short wynde. pluresis.

¶ also vryn rufe or subrufe w*ith* a mene body betwyn thycke. *and* thy*n*ne betokenyth a good dysposyssio*un* of helthe. //Gordian*us*.\\

¶ also vryn ruffe or s*u*bruffe in chyld //*and* thy*n*ne\\ betokenyth a ffeu*er* cotidian. //¶\\ and if it be more thycke þan thy*n*ne. and no skye nor dy*n*nesse above and the vryn apere so long tyme it betokenyth an hote dropsy. *and* aft*er* þ*a*t deth. //¶\\ ffor. theophile. seyth in his boke of vryns þ*a*t ruffe. *and* s*u*bruffe in þe d*r*opsye ys vncurabyl and white vryn i*n* þe d*r*opsye is good. *and* curabyl.

the hote dropsye. i*d est*. alchites. tympanytes. i*d est*. þe drye dropsy.

the Cold dropsye. i*d est*. yposarcha. leucofflewma.

¶ also vryn Ruffe or s*u*bruffe ou*er* all thycke. *and* dy*m*myssh above but not bloo þ*a*t is not moch dy*m*me betokenyth a ffeu*er* cotidian causyd of fflewm natural. Gordian*us*.

¶ also vryn Ruffe or s*u*bruffe w*ith* a

1431 Si…1433 coloris] *transp.* Debile rewm/a\tica me*m*bru*m* t*ur*bante qurela. Disponi pinguis pot*er*it rufi q*ue* coloris. Si spumosa mag*is* fiat cin*er*isq*ue* coloris. *m.r.* | **1433** poterit pinguis] *transp.* pinguis poterit *m.r.* | **1435** liuens] *corr. by exp.* //liuoris\\ *m.r.* | **1437** parum liuens] *corr. by exp.* and suprascr. parua liue*ns* *m.r.* | **1438** Obsita] *ins. by subscr.* i*d est*. plena *m.r.* | legata] *ins. by subscr.* i*d est* nuncia *m.r.*

1438 legata] Taken as *nuncia*, as in the note.

Rufe and subruf folow be order after citrin and is of mean colour betwen citrin and red s*ecundum* Io*hanem*. de. s*ancto*. a*mando*.

¶ themraud*is* dropsy. passi*ng* of flour*is*. fey*n*tnes of water tokneth stretnes at the brest and a feuer./
¶ a feu*er*. E*m*postym vnd*er* the ribbis. thartetic passio. short wynde. pluresis./

¶ Also vrin rufe /or\ subrufe with a mene bodi betwen thik and thin tokneth a good disposition of helth Gordianus.

¶ Rufe or subruf in childr*en* betokneth a feuer quotidian. and if it be more thik than thyn and no sky nor dymnes aboue on the vrin and the vrin apere so longe tyme it tokneth a hote dropsi and after that deth for teophile saith in his boke of vrins that Rufe and subruf in the dropsi is vncurable and white vrin in the dropsi is good and curable

¶ Alchytes. the hote dropsi

¶ Timpanites the dry dropsi

¶ Yposarcha ¶ leucoflegma the cold dropsy

¶ Also vrin Rufe or Subrufe ouer al thik and dy*m*mysh above but not bloo that is not moch Dym tokneth a feuer quo | tidian causid of fleume natural f. 9v
Gordianus

¶ Rufe or subrufe w*ith* a pure substance and equal betwyn thyn and thik in on that is sanguin it tokneth a good signe of helth Gordian*us*

¶ Rufe or subruf and thyn in wo*m*men that ben not sanguyn it tokneth a double tercian and in yong folk a feuer cotidian of fleume acetosu*m* and a simple tercian in old folke tha{t} ben fleumatik / and other

1160 rufe] *cancel.* and | **1177** Rufe] *cancel* and | **1184** sanguin] *cancel.* or subruf | **1190** that] *emend.* than

pure substance and equal betwyn thy*nn*e. *and* thicke in oon þ*a*t is sangueyn it betokenyth a good signe of helthe. Gordian*us*.

¶ also vryn Ruffe or *su*bruffe. *and* thy*n*ne. in wo*m*men þ*a*t ben | nat
f. 17v sangueyn it betokenyth a dobyl t*er*cian. //¶\\ and in yong ffolke a ffeu*er* cotidian of fflewm acetosu*m*. //¶\\ and a sympyl t*er*cian in olde ffolke þ*a*t ben fflewmatik. //¶\\ and oþ*er* sygnyficac*i*ons aft*er* þe co*n*tent*is* shew*n*. Galt*erius*.

¶ also in heruest yf it be long tyme aperyng sotyl *and* thy*n*ne and yardy. it betokenyth a quarteyn of col*er*. and of fflewm. *and* malencoly engendryd toged*er*. //¶\\ and oftyntymes it betokenyth skaldyng of þe. lyu*er*. throwght outragi*us* hetis ayens kynde. Galt*erius*. *and* Egidi*us*.

¶ also vryn. Ruffe or *su*bruffe menely thicke or menely thy*n*ne w*ith* a man*er* of bloones. above. and grene it betokenyth þe sp*irit*ual me*m*brys be hurt w*ith* moch plente of salt fflewm. and þe cough. *and* streytnes of breth. and dyssesyd at þe breste. //¶\\ and it nat cloudy of long tyme w*ith* greynys above it betokenyth þe hote d*r*opsy. *and* aft*er* þ*a*t to dye //¶\\ and it be of þe ffeu*er* of salt fflewm it is w*ith* g*re*te drynes *and* saltnes of þe mowth. *and* w*ith* st*r*ong peyne in þe hed. and sornes in the butokk*is* &. silia*m*. Egidi*us*. Gilb*er*t*us*. Galt*erius*.

¶ and if such vryn apere w*ith* many smale resoluc*i*ons w*ith* a man*er* of bloones and grene it betokenyth moch. plente of wynde. *and* of scabys. Egidi*us*. ysaac.

¶ also such vryn betokenyth in wo*m*men peyne i*n* her*e* mat*r*ice. anamely vnd*er* her*e* lefftte syde walwyng. *and* ffretyng. *and* w*ith* vnkynde fylth of þe mat*r*ice it is for t*ra*ueyld *and* swoln w*ith* hurlyng. *and* worchyn of dyu*er*se hum*er*s. and moch wynd /w*ith*\ swellyng. *and* penawnce of her*e* p*r*ivy me*m*b*er*. Gord*ianus*.

¶ also such vryn betokenyth þe ffeu*er*

significations after the contentes shewed Galteri*us*

¶ Also in hervest if it be long tyme appering sotel and thyn and yardy it betokneth a quarteyn of coler and of flewme and melancoli engendred together and often tymes it tokneth scalding of the lyuer thorow owtragious hetis ayenst kinde Galteri*us* Egidius

¶ Rufe or subrufe menly {thik} or menly thyn w*ith* a maner of blones above and grene it tokneth the spiritual membres be hurt w*ith* moch plente of salt flewm. and the cough and streitnesse of breth and diseased at the brest and it not clowdy of longe tyme w*ith* greynys ¶ above it tokneth the hote dropsy and after that to dy ¶ and it be of salt flewm it is w*ith* great drynesse and saltnesse of the mouth and w*ith* strong payn in the hede and sornesse of the bottok*is*. et silia*m* Egidius. Gilbert*us*. Galterius

¶ And if souch vrin appere w*ith* many smal resolutions w*ith* a maner of blones and grene it tokneth moch plenty of winde and of scabbes Egidi*us*. Ysaac.

¶ Such vrin in women /tokneth\ payn in here matrice and namely vnder her lift side waluyng and freting w*ith* vnkind hete and filthe of the matrice it is for trauel and swolni*ng* w*ith* hurling and working of diuerse humoures and moche wind and swelling and penaunce of her prevy membre Gordian*us*.

¶ Also souch an vrin tokneth a fever Emit*r*iceus w*ith* breding of a postym vnd*er* the brest that is called pleure*sis* w*ith* priking vnd*er* the ribbis above the mydrif or els p*er*lyleumo*n*ia that is an empostem vnd*er* both the sides w*ith* rednes of the Iawes of the mydrif vpwarde to the lunges and in the lung*is* and the hert is evil at ease, and (but god help) it is but deth And whan it is of peripleumo*n*ia the vryn is more thynner and louer of c{o}lour than whan it war of pleuresis. Egid*ius*.

1515 of[1]] *cancel.* w*ith*

1505 dropsy] *ext. marg.* d*ropsy* | **1518** wommen] *ext. marg.* mulier

1195 appering] *rep.* appering | **1204** tokneth] *cancel.* a quarte*i*n | **1234** perlyleumonia] *cancel.* phylo | **1242** it] *cancel.* is

¶ A ffeu*er* corruptt. *and* blood of a veyn brokyn in þe back. and þe fflourys.

¶ also red colo*ur* is more hiȝer. *and* depper þan is Ruffe colo*ur*. it is a mene colour*e* betwyn Red go/l\d and Red blood. /it\ is causyd of blood. and of Col*er* megtt toged*er*. ypoc*ras*. & Egidi*us*.

¶ and if it be thicke. *and* tr*o*bly it stondyth be blood. and yf it be bryȝtt. *and* clere. it stondyth be coler. ypoc*ras*.

¶ also vryn rubea or subrube/a\ mor*e* //thicke\\ above þan benethe with a dy*m*nes. above. it hayth dyu*er*se signyficacio*u*ns upon dyu*er*se agys. and dyu*er*se *com*plexio*u*ns. ffor in a chylde it betokenyth a ffeu*er* cotidian. and in yong ffolke anamely of colryk *com*plexio*u*n is a //sy*m*pil\\ t*er*cian and in olde ffolke anamely i*n* fflewmatyk or male*n*coly. it is a dobyl t*er*cian. Egidi*us*. auic*enna*. ysaac.

¶ also in wo*m*men *and* pr*in*cipaly yf þe maledy haue nat lastyd long. as but. a day. or. ij. or. iij. þan it betokenyth a dobyl t*er*cian. Egidi*us*. auyce*nna*.

f. 19v ¶ also Red vryn all thy*n*ne. *and* cler*e*. *and* shadwyd above *and* gretly ȝardy above w*ith* smale greynes it betokenyth a ffeu*er* quarteyn w*ith* peyne in þe ryȝtt syde. and wyth hardenes of þe splen. Egidi*us*. & Ioh*anes* de s*an*cto *am*ando.

¶ and if it be thy*n*ne and shadwyd. above. *and* w*ith* a yelo spwme þan the peyne is in þe ryȝtt syde and if it haþ be so long. *and* no ffeu*er*. it is caleffaccio*u*n of þe lyu*er*. Egidi*us*.

¶ also an vryn menely thicke. *and* tr*o*bly and equal in s*u*bsta*u*nce betokenyth a *con*tinval t*er*cian of col*er* put*ri*fied in the grete veynes. Egidi*us*.

¶ also vryn may be made thicke. *and* tr*o*bly. in. iij. man*er* wysys. somtyme it is thicke because of nobyl

1629 blood[1]] *cancel.* the | **1636** more] *cancel.* thynne

1626 red] *int. marg.* Red colo*ur* | **1628** mene] *ext. marg.* c*om*plexio | **1647** wommen] *ext. marg.* mulier t*er*cian | **1669** also] *ext. marg.* Rew*le* | **1670** somtyme] *ext. marg.* .i.

and clere it stondeth be coler Ypoc*ras*.

¶ Rubea or subrubea more thik above than bineþe w*ith* dymnes above it hath diuerse significations vpon diuerse agis and diuerse c*om*plexions for in a child it tokneth a feuer | cotidian and f. 10v
in yong folk and namely of colerik complexion it is a simple tercian and in olde folk and nameli in flewmatik or malencoly it is a dowble tercian Egidi*us* Auic*enna* Ysaac.

¶ Also in women and principaly if the maledy haue not lasted long as but a day or ij or iij than it tokneth a dowble tercyan Egid*ius*. auic*enna*

¶ Red vrin and /al\ thyn and clere and shadowed above greatly yardy above w*ith* smal greynes it tokneth a fever quarte*in* w*ith* payn in the right side and hardnesse of the splene Egid*ius*. & Io*hanem* de s*ancto* a*mando*.

¶ And if it be thyn and shadowed above w*ith* a yelow spume than the payn is on the right side. and if it hath be so long and no feuer it is calefaction of the lyuer Egid*ius*.

¶ Also vrin may be made thik and trobly in thre man*er* ways su*m*tyme it is thik bicawse of noble digestion but than it is but litil thik w*ith* a clerenesse and a brightnesse in coloure that is /a\ good {token} for that tokneth that he is myty in kinde, and su*m*tym because the vrin is thik because of feblenesse, and be largenesse, and wey of the vryn. and if it be feblenes of kinde therin is p*er*el ffor it is a tokyn that kind is not of power in hymself to w*ith*stonde ne to kepe in the body the humoures, and su*m*tym it is thik because of multitude and distemp*er* of su*m* humor or of su*m* humours but /in\ both the ij last poynt*is* the vrin is more thik and more ded in colo*ur* than whan it is thik because of good digestio*un* Eg*idius*. Ysa*ac*. Auic*enna*.

¶ Red and meanely thik above w*ith* grenesh spume and w*ith* the co*n*tent Attemose hanging in the mydd*is* and su*m*what grenysh tokneth moch

1314 complexions] *ext. marg.* c*om*plexio

dygestio*u*n. but than it is but litell thicke w*ith* a clernes. *and* a bryhtnesse in colo*ur* þ*at* is a good tokyn ffor it betokenyth þ*at* he is myȝty in kynde. // and somtyme because þe vryn is thicke be ffebyl/nes\ of kynde and be largenesse. *and* wey of þe vryn. and yf it be be ffebylnes of kynde þ*er*in is p*er*el. for it is a tokyn þ*at* kynde is nat of power*e* i*n* hi*m*selff to w*ith*stonde ne to kepe /in\ the body þe hum*er*s. // and somtyme it is thicke because of multytud. *and* dystemp*er* of som humo*ur* or of som hum*er*s. but in b/o\the these. ij. last poyntis þe vry*n* is mor*e* thycke *and* mor*e* ded i*n* colo*ur* þan whan it is thick because of good digestio*u*n. Egidi*us*. ysaac. auic*enna*.

¶ also vryn red. *and* menely thicke. *and* liȝtt above w*ith* a grenysh spume. *and* w*ith* þe *con*te*n*te attemose hangy*n*g in the mydys. *and* somewhatt

f. 20r grenysh betokenyth | moch mat*er* aduste. and a postym þ*at* is callyd plurecis and þan þe vryn is grenysh or yelwysh *and* wa*n*nysh above. s*ecundu*m. Egidi*um*. & Ioh*anem*. de. *sancto*. a*mando*.

¶ also vryn rube*us* or s*u*brube*us* passyng thy*n*ne w*ith* a g*r*ene cerkyl it betoken*yth* moch wickyd sykens of col*er*. *secundum*. Gilb*ertum*. li*bro*. p*rimo*. ca*pitulo*. p*rimo*. de t*er*ciana. //¶\\ and if it be rube*us* w*ith* a sharpe syknes it is bett*er* þan it wer*e*. a white watry colo*ur*. auicen*na*. ca*pitulo* p*rimo*.

¶ also Red vryn w*ith* sor*e* syknes i*n* þe back. pessi*ma* e*st*. for it betokenyth an hott postym in þe back. *and* yf it be w*ith* strong peyne in þe hed it is nat so evyl. auic*enna*. ca*pitul*o. p*rimo*.

¶ and if it be red. *and* trobly. *and* onywhile so *con*tynuy*n*g it betokenyth a postym in þe lyu*er*. *and* hardnes þ*er*of. auic*enna*. p*rimo*.

¶ also vryn Rube*us* þe wech is somwhat blackysh it betokenyth a ffeu*er com*pounyd. and if it be black vpward and þe vr/yn\ cler*e* þan it betokenyth. a postym i*n* þe sydis. auicen*na*.

¶ also vryn red. *and* thicke. *and* grose

1676 somtyme] *ext. marg.* .2. | **1684** somtyme] *ext. marg.* .3.

matter aduste and a postym that is called pleuresis and than the vryn is grenysh or yelowesh a{nd} wa*n*nysh above. Egid*ium* & Io*hanem*. d*e*. *sancto*. a*mando*.

¶ Red or subred passing thyn w*ith* a grene cerkil it tokneth moch wiked siknesse of Coler s*ecundu*m Gilbertu*m* l*ibr*o. ca*pitul*o p*rim*o de terciana and it be rubea w*ith* a sharp siknesse is better than it wer a white watri colour Auic*enna* ca*pitulo*. p*rim*o.

¶ Red vrin w*ith* sore siknesse in the bak pessima est ffor it tokneth a hote postym in the bak and if it be w*ith* a strong peyn in the hede it is not so evil Auic*enna* ca*pitulo* p*rim*o.

¶ Red and trobly eny while so *con*tynuyng it tokneth a {postym} in the lyu*er* and hardnesse therof

¶ Red which is su*m*what blakysh it tokneth a feuer co*m*powند and if it be blac vpwarde and the vrin cler*e* than it tokneth a postym in the sides Auic*enna*.

¶ Red vrin and thik {and} grose w*ith* drynesse in the rofe of the mowth and bitternesse therin and stynking w*ith* synging in ther erys tokneth great hete. and litil rest sheding of mouch sond and brent bloode in the lyuer and great perel Auic*enna*. 4°.

¶ Red fatty and grose and thre | f. 11r
ypostasis daily shyning tokneth sharp siknesse of Sinochis Auic*enna*

¶ Red and fatty and litil w*ith* drynesse in the mowth therin is p*er*el w*ith* defnesse and ache in the hede, in the nec, and in the right side and the iaund*is* and deth on the 7 day Ptolom*eus*.

¶ Red with fayr white ypostas*is* tokneth warishing of the siknesse, and if it be red and lite it tokneth the artetica passio and alienation of mynd Ysaac and if it be red and sotil pessima e*st* Yssac

¶ Red w*ith* blac ypostas*is* and

1387 and[2]] *emend.* w*ith*

w*ith* drynesse in the roffe of þe mowthe. *and and* bitternesse þerynne. *and* stynckyng w*ith* synggyng of þe Erys betokenyth grete hete. *and* lytell reste shedyng of moch seed. *and* brentt blood in þe lyu*er*. *and* gr*o*se p*er*el. auicen*na*. 4º.

¶ vryn s*u*brubeu*s* fatty. *and* grosse. and þe ypostasis dayly shyny*ng* betokenyth sharpe sykenes as sinochus. auic*enna*.

¶ and if it be red. *and* fatty. *and* lytel w*ith* drynesse i*n* the mowthe þery*n*ne is p*er*el. w*ith* deffnes. and ach in the hed. and i*n* þe necke. *and* in þe ryȝtt

f. 20v syde. *and* | the Iawndys. *and* deth. on þe. 7 day. theo*philu*s.

¶ vryn red w*ith* ffayr white ypostasis betokenyth warysshyng of þe sykenes. and if it /be\ red *and* lyȝtt it betokenyth þe artetyca passio. *and* alyenacio*u*n of mynde. ysaac. and if it be red. *and* sotyl. pessi*m*a e*st*. yssac.

¶ also vryn red w*ith* black ypostasis. *and* stynkyng and trobly. *and* as it wer*e* herys it is wickyd *and* deth. ypoc*ra*s.

¶ and if it be red wi*th*out ypostasis betokenyth ffaylyng of natur*e* *and* an hote feu*er*. & pessi*m*a e*st*. ysaac.

¶ also vryn red. *and* gr*o*se nat shyny*ng* w*ith* peyne in þe Erys. and in þe hed. and in þe riȝtt syde it betokenyth þe Iawndys pessi*m*a e*st*. ysaac.

¶ vryn red and gr*o*se i*n* a sharpe ffeu*er* it betokenyth eu*er* peyne in þe hed. *and* i*n* þe nekke. and in the ryȝtt syde. ypoc*ra*s. ysaac.

¶ also vryn red as wyn. or blood wi*th*out peyne in þe hed it betokenyth dayly labo*ur*. and if it *con*tinue it betokenyth sykenes in þe bladd*er*. ypoc*ra*s.

¶ and if it {be} red as blod in a sharpe ffeu*er* it betokenyth sodeyn deth. ypoc*ra*s.

¶ also Red vryn w*ith* þe Iawndys. *and* somwhatt whitysh it betokenyth peyne in the hed. and alyenacio*u*n of mynde. ypoc*ra*s.

¶ also vryn red. w*ith* spuyng and sharpnes of þe tung it betokenyth deth. ypoc*ra*s.

stinking and trobly as it war heris it is wicked and deth Ypoc*ra*s.

¶ Red wi*th*out yposta*sis* tokneth failing of nature and an hote feuer et pessi*m*a est Ysaac

¶ Red and grose not shyni*ng* w*ith* peyn in the Eris and in the hede and in the right side it tokneth the Iaund*is* pessi*m*a est Ysaac

¶ Red and grose in a sharp feu*er* it tokneth eu*er* payn in the hede and in the nec, and in the right side Ypoc*ras* Ysaac

¶ Red as wyn or blood wi*th*out payn in the hede it tokneth daily labour and if it contynow it tokneth siknesse in the bladd*er* Ypoc*ras*.

¶ And if it be red as blod in a sharp feuer it tokneth soden deth Ypoc*ras*

¶ Red vrin w*ith* the iaund*is* and su*m*what whitesh it tokneth great peyn in the hede and alienation of mynde Ypocras

¶ Red vrin w*ith* spuyng and sharpnes of the tunge it tokneth dethe Ypoc*ras*

¶ Red as blode in a sharp feuer tokneth dethe. and namely if he haue gret drede at the hart and pein in the right side

¶ Be he ware of al indigest met*is* and diet hym w*ith* such as shal gender and norish good humors as poork and flesh of yong best*is*. and chykyns and fish of swete wateres and oximel and cassiafistula and tisannys &c

Take the ius of moleyn and of hartistong and of watercres*sis* and verveyn isop beteyn wormode triacle sethe al these in white wyn and d*rink* *and* p*roba*.

//¶\\ and it be red as blood i*n* a sh*a*rpe
f. 21r ffeu*er*. sig*nificat* morte*m*. anamely if | he haue g*r*ete drede at þe h*er*te. *and* peyne i*n* þe riȝtt syde

¶ Be he whar*e* of all indigest met*is*. and diete hi*m* w*ith* such as shall gend*er*. *and* norysh good hum*er*s. as porke. *and* fflesh of yong best*is*. and Chikenes. and ffyssh of swete watrys *and* oximel. and cassia fistula and tysa*n*nys. &c

Take the Iuce of moleyn. *and* of h*er*t*is*tung. *and* of wat*er*cressis. *and* v*er*veyne. ysope. beteyn. wormde. and t*r*iacle. sethe all these. i*n* white wyn. *and* d*r*y*nk*. *and*. p*r*o*ba*.

CErcior est testis Rubicu*n*di fforma coloris.

. Rubicu*n*dus.
¶ a ffeuer acute ou*er* sett at þe h*er*te *and* deffawt of wynde. ¶ the rewme i*n* þe hed. deffnes. pose *and* hevynes.

¶ Rubicu*n*da is moste hiȝest in colo*ur* þ*at* is or may be. it is most lyke to red blood or to a ffynne red rose þ*at* is briȝtt. *and* ffressh. and subrubicu*n*de is moste like to wat*er*blood or ell*is* to a rose þ*at* is deffadyd of his colo*ur* //or fflawme of ffyre.\\ s*ecundu*m. ysaac.

¶ also vnd*er*stond this for a gene*r*al reule that what vryn so eu*er* it be if it thicke. *and* cler*e* hy*m*selffe above. and
f. 21v yf þ*at* thicknes drawe down | to the Resydence in þe botym. and it waxyt thy*n*ne and Cler*e* aboue. sig*nificat* warysshyng of þe maledy. ysaac.

¶ and yf þe vryn be clere benethe and thicke aboue it betokenyth deth. ysaac.

¶ also if þe vryn be red. *and* stynkyth w*ith* black ypostasis. *and* t*r*obly. and hath bodyes lyke herys or ell*is* lyke scurffe or bran {it betokenyth} //excesse of digesty*ou*n. *and* also adusty*ou*n. ysaac.\\ {et} sig*nifica*t. morte*m*. ysaac.

¶ also vryn Rubicu*nd*. *and*. s*u*brubicu*nd*. thicke. *and* nat wanysh aboue. *and* somdel g*r*enysh

Rubicu*ndus*
a feu*er* acute ov*er*set at the h*er*te and defawte of wynde. Rewme in the hede. defnes. pose and hevynes.

Rubicunde is most hiest in colour that is or may be it is most like vnto red blode, or to a fyne red rose that is very clere and bright and fresh ¶ and Subrubicund is most like to water bloode. or els to a rose that is defadid of his colour or flawm of fir*e* Ysaac.

¶ Also vnd*er*stond | this for a general f. 11v
rule that what vrin it be and if it thik and clere hymself above and if that thiknesse drawe down to the residens in the botom and waxeth thyn and clere above sig*nifica*t warishing of the maledi Ysaac

¶ And if the vrin be cler*e* and thik above it tokneth deth Ysaac

Also if þe vrin be red and stynketh w*ith* blac yposta*sis* and hath bodies like heris or scurf*is* or bran it tokneth excesse of digestion and also adustion Ysaac et sig*nifica*t morte*m* Ysaac

¶ Rubicu*n*de or subrubycunde thik and not wa*n*nysh above and su*m*dele grenysh tokneth a feuer sinothica. which is engendred of blood in the reynes or els sinocha that is a co*n*tynual feuer Egidius. Ysa*ac*.

And this vrin be thyn and bright and clere it tokneth a feuer causon or synochiden the which is engendred of moch colerik matter w*ith* the

1804 and[2]] *cancel.* Ru

1785 diete] *ext. marg.* dieta | **1791** Take] *ext. marg.* medicina | **1796** coloris] ext. marg. *versus*

¶ also such an vryn in a ffeu*er* betokenyth waryssHsyng þe bledyng at þe nose. //.ysaac.\\

f. 23r ¶ these colou*res* in wo*m*men. somtyme it betokenyth a ffeu*er*. *and* somtyme syknes of her*e* fflour*is*. but whan it is of þe fflourys þe vryn is mor*e* thick *and* t*ro*bly downward þan whan it is of a ffeu*er*. *and* is eue*r*more suspeckt in men þan in wo*m*man. ypoc*ras*.

¶ also vryn. y*n*nopos. or kyanos w*ith* mykel resydence in a wo*m*man þ*at* hath not her*e* fflourys it betokenyth warysshyng be brestyng out of þe fflourys. theo*philus*.

¶ also yf þ*er* be oneþys ony resydence i*n* þe botym of þe vrynal or ell*is* noo*n*. yf she be t*ra*ueyled w*ith*. a ffeu*er*. *and* haþ not her*e* fflour*is* it betokenyth deth. Egidi*us*.

¶ the same wyse in a man of þe emrawdys yf þe emrawdys be stoppyd. *and* re*n*ne nat morte*m* sig*nifica*t. Egidi*us*.

¶ also vryn ynnopos or kyanos þ*at* hath no resyde*n*ce in þe botym in man or wo*m*man. morte*m* sig*nifica*t. Egidi*us*.

¶ also it betokenyth þ*at* dyue*rs* hum*ers* in þe body ben so wyckyd. or so Corrupt þ*at* it is impossibyle þ*at* kynde shuld oue*r*com hem or for to mayst*ri* hem. and þ*er*for in such sykenes þe pacyent is nat for to take i*n* honde. //Gilb*ertus*.\\

¶ also vryn ynnopos betokenyth pyssyng of blood and somtyme þ*at* þe veynes be brokyn þ*at* comyn from þe kyl/e\ veyne. and somtyme. a postem of þe blood in þe lyu*er*. *and* than þ*at* pyssyng stynkyth nat. Egidi*us*.

¶ also y*n*nopos somtyme betokenyth a bre*n*ny*n*g hum*er* in þe reynes. and that þe lyu*er* is forscaldyd w*ith* bredy*n*g of þe Iawndis. and þe hote d*ro*psy. Egidi*us*.

¶ also yf it be t*ro*bly in þe botu*m* mor*e*
f. 23v þan ell*is* wher*e* it | betokenyth brestyng of som veyne. or of excesse of lechery. *and* than þ*er* apere ropyng

¶ Ynopos or kianos w*ith* mekil residens in a woman that hath not her floures it tokneth warishing to bresting owt of the floures Ptolom*eus*

¶ Also if ther be onethis ony resydens in the botom of the vrinal or els non if she be traueld w*ith* a feuer and hath not her flour*is* it tokneth dethe Egidi*us* /

¶ The same wise in a man in the Emeraud*is* if the emerawd*is* be stopped *and* renne nat morte*m* Egid*ius*.

¶ Ynopos or kianos that hath no residens in the botom in man or woman morte*m* sig*nifica*t Egid*ius*

¶ Also it tokneth that diuerse humours in the body ben so wicked and so corrupt that it is vnpossible that kind shuld oue*r*cu*m* him or for to mast*er* hym and therfor in souch siknes the pacient is not for to take in hand Gilbert*us*

¶ Ynopos tokneth pissing of bloode and sumtym that the veynes be broke that cu*m*yth fro*m* the kilis veyn, and su*m*tym an empostym of the blood in the lyver, and than that pissing styngketh not Egid*ius*.

¶ Also ynopos su*m*tym tokneth a bre*n*nyng humour in the reynes and that the lyver is forscalded w*ith* breding of the Iaund*is* and the hote dropsy Egidius

Also if it be trobly in the botom mor than elswher it tokneth bresting of
su*m* veyn | or of exesse of lechery and f. 12v
than ther apereth roping thing*is* or white glete or sp*er*me and long resolutions red and raw it is an evil signe both in kianos and in ynopos Gilbert*us*

Also it tokneth the ston and the colik and pleure*sis* and empostym vnd*er* the right side above the mydrif w*ith* streytnesse of winde and moch penans at tharte and in the reynes a feble stomok thorow overpassing of digestion than the vrin is nygh like to sinop and betokneth deth Gilbert. et Io*hanem*. de. *sancto*. a*mando*.

1962 kyl/e\] *cancel.* kyl~~ys~~

1926 wommen] *ext. marg.* *mulier*

1602 tokneth] *cancel.* bl

thyng*is* or white glett. or sp*er*me. *and* long resoluc*i*ons red *and* rawe. *and* it is an evyl signe boþe i*n* kyanos or i*n* y*n*nopos. Gilb*ertus*.

¶ also it betokenyth þe ston. and þe Colik. *and* pluresis. and. a postem vnd*er* þe Ryȝtt syde. above þe mydryff w*ith* streytnes of wynde. *and* moch penawnce at the herte. *and* i*n* þe reynes. a ffebyl stomak throwh ouerpassyng of dygestio*un* þan þe vryn is nyȝh lyke to Synop. and betokenyth deth. Gilb*ertus*. &. Iohanes. de s*an*cto *a*mando.

¶ also vryn y*n*nopos. or kyanos w*ith* a *cont*/i\nual ffeu*er* or yf it aper*e* black. *and* moch in qua*n*tyte. w*ith* good sig*n*is of digestyo*un* þan þ*er* is hope of recur*e*. and yf it ffayle good signys of digestion it betoken*yth* hasty deþ. //Walt*erius*. Egidi*us*.\\

¶ vryn y*n*nopos lytel. *and* thicke w*ith* black ypostasis malu*m* sig*nifica*t. *and* betokenyth a postem in þe reynes and if it be thicke. *and* lyȝhtt above. and shadwyd w*ith* a yelwe spwme it betokenyth an hote postem in the lyu*er*. Egidi*us*. & Galt*erius*.

¶ and if it be thicke benethe it betokenyth the Emrawdys or þe fflourys. Egidi*us*.

¶ and if it com in an hole body w*ith* a thicke substa*u*nce *and* bloodylyke betokenyth brekyng of som veyne w*ith* skyppyng or goyng or ou*er*moch*e* takyng luste of wo*m*men. Galt*erius*. & Egidi*us*. & Gilb*ertus*. //¶\\ and yelwe spwme in a wo*m*man betoken*yth* rete*n*cion of fflouris. ysaac.

f. 24r ¶ also yf kyanos apere w*ith* wyndy *con*tentys it betokenyth grete hurte in þe bladd*er*. and pusshys. and þe st*ra*nguryon anamely yf it be in holde ffolke w*ith* peyne *and* p*r*ickyng i*n* þe fflankys. //yssac.\\

The signys /of\ hem. moch thrust. *and* moch swellyng before mete. and onlusty to do onythyng but eu*er* sloggy. *and* hevy.

1991 hope] *cancel.* ope | **2011** spwme] *cancel.* spwma

1982 herte] *ext. marg.* adustion | **2014** kyanos] *top. marg.* a bre*n*nyng ffeu*er* in þe body | **2020** signys] *ext. marg.* Signa

¶ Ynapos or kianos w*ith* a co*n*tinual feuer or if it appere blac and moche in quantite w*ith* goode synys of digestion than ther is hope of recover and if it fail good synes of digestion it tokneth hasty deth W*alterius*. Egid*ius*.

¶ Ynopos litil and thik w*ith* blac ipostasis malu*m* sig*nifica*t and tokneth a postym in the reynes and if it be thik and lite above and shadowed w*ith* a yelo spume it tokneth a hote postym in the lyuer Egid*ius*. Galter*ius*.

¶ And if it be thik beneth it tokneth the emerawd*is* or the flouris Egid*ius*.

and if it cum in an hole body w*ith* a thik substans and blodylike it tokneth breking of sum veyn w*ith* scipping or goyng or overmoch taki*n*g lust of women Galter*ius* Egid*ius*. Gilb*ertus*. and yelo spume in a woman tokneth retention of here flourys Ysaac.

Also if kianos apere w*ith* windy content*es* it betokneth great hurt in the bladder and pushes, and the strangurion and namely if it be in old folk w*ith* payn and prikking in the flankis Yssac

¶ The synes of hem moch thurst and moch swelling bifore and vnlusty to do enything but ever sluggy and hevy

¶ Thow shalt dyet hym fro*m* met*is* of indigestion As porret*is* wortis al salt met*is* and met*is* that ben fat

¶ Take spineg*e* Columby*n* turme*n*tyl matfelon. and the sed of fumytere and of gold*is* of eche an handful and drye hem out of the sun and make therof poud*er* and vse it

¶ Another pre febre ¶ Take wormode Rue herb benet Dandelion and mercury p*er*sly rotis fenel rot*is* borage violett*is* saturyon vineger Licor*is* triacle the Ius of sorel and piliol mownteyn al this compounde and soden in ale or white wyn and vse it to drink yerly and Late

¶ Item ¶ Take Osmu*n*d Saven Gromel Endyve Liuerwort setwhale Oculus *Christ*i purified hony white hony and so compou*n*d

¶ Thou shalt diet him from metis of Indigestion as porrettis. wortis all salt metis. *and* metis þat ben ffatte. &c

Take Spynegre. Columbyn. turmentyl. matfelon. *and* the sed of ffumitterre. *and* of Goldys of ech. a handfful. *and* drye hem out of þe sonne. *and* make þerof pouder and vse it.

anoþer. per ffebre. Take. wormode. Rue. herbe benet. dawndelyon. *and* mercurye. persly rotis. ffenel rotis. borage. vyolettis. satirion. veneger. licoryis. triacle. *and* þe Iuce of sorel. *and* pylliol mownteyn. all this. compounyd. *and* sodyn in ale or white wyn. *and* vsyd to be drunkyn erly. *and* late.

¶ anoþer. take. Osmu{n}tt. Saveyn. gromyle. Endyve. lyuerwortt. setwale. oculus *Christi*. puryfied hony. *and* white wyn. //*and* so compounyd.\\

. Grene. colour.

¶ þe krampe. wynde. vanyte in þe hed. ¶ þe morfu. empostymmys. þe gowtte.

¶ also grene colour betokenyth euer adustion. auicenna. primo. ¶ also grene vryn betokenyth þe Iawnys. and þer ben. iij. maner of. Iawnys the. i.
f. 24v spice is lest malicious | and is best to hele. and it is clepyd. icterìcia glauca. the. 2. spice is callyd pegaselen. i*d est*. mustela agrestis. or agriacam. or icterìcia viridis. an whan þe vryn is lyke grene gresse it betokenyth deth.// the. 3. spice is cl/e\pyd in gru melanchimon. in laten melanchina. i*d est*. icterìcia nigra. þat is a swart grene lyke marubium þat is horehounde. & pessima. est. aueroi. 4º.

¶ also grene vryne in an agu betokenyth a maledy þat is clepyd Spasmus. i*d est*. þe Crampe // and Thetanus. is clepyd þe shote./ and þerfor. ysodore seyth in the. iiij. boke of Ethymologies. þe. vj. chapter. þat

2024 diet] *ext. marg.* dieta | **2027** Take] *ext. marg.* medicina | **2053** icterìcia glauca] ext. marg. þe yelw Iawnys | **2054** 2] *ext. marg.* .2. | **2056** icterìcia viridis] *ext. marg.* þe grene Iawnys | **2058** 3] *ext. marg.* .3. | **2060** icterìcia nigra] *ext. marg.* þe black Iawnys | **2066** Crampe] *ext. marg.* þe Crampe | **2067** shote/] *ext. marg.* þe shote | **2068** ysodore] *ext. marg.* Rewle

the cramp. wind. vanite in thede. the morfew. Empostems. the gout

ALSO GRENE colour betokneth ever adustion Auicenna primo. Also grene vrin tokneth the Iaundis ¶ And ther be iij maner of Iaundis ¶ The first spice is lest malicious. and is best to hele. and is cleped Ictericia glauca the yelo Iawndis ¶ The 2 spice is called phegaselem. i*d est*. muste | la agrestis f. 13r
or agriacam or ictericia viridis. And whan the vrin is like grene gras it tokneth deth ¶ The iij[d] spice is clepid in grew melanchimon in laten melanchinia. i*d est*. ictericia nigra that is a swart gren like marrubium that is horhownd et pessima est Aueroi 4

¶ Also grene vryn in an agu tokneth a maledy that is callid spasmus. i*d est* the crampe, and Tetanus is clepid the shote And therfor Ysodorus saith in the fourth boke of Ethimologies vjº capitulo. That Spasmus is the lesse contraction of partise in the body comyng sodenly in the synows with houg payn caused of replecion of wiked humours in the synows, and

1681 in²] *cancel.* me

1681 melanchimon] *ext. marg.* me lanchimon | **1690** Spasmus] *ext. marg.* spasmus spasme is þe lesse *contra*cciou*n* of p*ar*ties in þe body co*m*myng sodenly in þe senuys w*ith* hoge peyne causyd of replecion of wyckyd hum*er*s i*n* þe senuys. and somtyme it comyth of a ventysshyng of kyndly hete in the senuys. Th/e\tan*us* is þe more spasm*us*. and it is causyd of *con*supciou*n* of þe kyndly substancy/a\l humydite in the body.

¶ also grene vryn þ*at* is lytel betokenyth deth. anamely if it stynke or yf it barke or bleche þe a place þ*er* it is leyd on. auycen*na*. p*rimo*.

¶ also grene vryn. *and* mykel i*n* qua*n*tyte *and* it stynke not nor barke not. *and* þ*er*w*ith* his ache is good þan þ*er* is hope of lyfe. auycen*na*. //¶\\ and as it is reersyd afore of lytel vryn *and*
f. 25r grene. so it is to b*e* vnd*er* | stonde in blacke colo*ur*. *and* in bloo colo*ur* as well as in grene colour. auycen*na*.

¶ also gre*n* vryn. *and* moch. *and* moddy. w*ith* an evyl sauo*ur* betokenyth p*ar*brakyng and blemsshyng of som nobyl me*m*b*er* in þe body. *and* the substancyall humydite of þ*at* me*m*b*er* passyth awey w*ith* þe vryn and betokenyth hasty deth. auycen*na*.

¶ also grene vryn betokenyth the morffu. *and* vanyte in þe hed. w*ith* grete akthe. and if it be grene in an agu it betokenyth þe krampe at h*er*te w*ith* wastyng of þe s*u*bstancyal moystnes. Gilb*ertus*.

¶ also if it be but of his p*r*opyr colo*ur* it betokenyth. a postem i*n* þe stomak. Gilb*ertus*.

¶ also if it be somwhat g*r*enysh. *and* swart. *and* moch in qua*n*tyte it betokenyth þe mor*e*. Emit*r*iceus w*ith*y*n*ne þe veynes. *and* coler w*ith*out. and it is eu*er* bre*n*ny*n*g. *and* scaldyng *and* deth. auic*enna*.

¶ also grene colour as it were grene oyle havyng a cloude of þe eyr*e* w*ith* strong savour betokenyth consu*m*pciou*n* and aft*er* þ*at* deth. auicen*na*. & ysaac. vnde dic*it* galyen. Si vnctositas *consu*m*pcione*ȝ pingueis sig*nifica*t. & om*n*i me*m*bror*um*

2107 betokenyth] *del.* and

su*m*tym it comyth of a ventishing of kindly hete in the synows ¶ Thetan*us* is the more spasm*us* and is cawsed of consumption of the kindly substantial humydite in the body

¶ Also vrin that is litil tokneth deth and namely if it stink or if it barke or blech the a place ther it is leid on Auic*enna* p*rimo*

¶ Grene vrin and mykil in quantite and it stink not nor bark not and therw*ith* his age is good than ther is hope of lif Auic*enna* And as it is rehersed afore of litil vryn and gren so it is to be vnd*er*stand in blac colour and in blo colour as wel as in gren colo*ur* Auic*enna*

¶ Also grene vrin and moch and modly w*ith* an evil sauour tokneth p*ar*braking and blemishing of su*m* noble membre in the body and the substantialle humydite of that membre passeth away w*ith* the vrin and tokneth hasty deth Auic*enna*

Also grene vrin tokneth the morfew and vanyte in thede w*ith* great akith and if it be greyn In an agu it tokneth the cramp at the hert w*ith* wasting of the substantial moistnesse Gilbert*us*

¶ Also if it be but of his propir colour it tokneth an empostym in the stomok Gilbert*us*

¶ Also su*m*what gre*n*nysh and swart and moch in qua*n*tite it tokneth the more Emitrice*us* w*ith*in the veynes and coler w*ith*out, and it is ever bre*n*ni*n*g and scalding and deth auic*enna*

¶ Also gren colour as it war gren oil having a cloud of the eyer w*ith* strong sauour betokneth co*n*su*m*ption and after that deth auic*enna*. Ysa*ac*. vnde dicit gal*en*. Si vnctositas co*n*su*m*pcio*nem* pingueis sig*nifica*t et o*mn*i membro*rum* duro*rum* Et Eruginosa peior est & pentile*n*cior qu*am* vnctuosa & fuit pessie*m*

1705 stink] *cancel.* a

1696 Thetanus] *ext. marg.* thetanus | 1719 morfew] *ext. marg.* morfew | 1735 consumption] *ext. marg.* Co*n*su*m*ptiou*n*

Hinc Ipocr*as* veri semina vera t*r*ahit.
//¶\\ Nu*n*c contentor*um* seriatim forma notet*ur*.
Et tenea*n*t p*r*oprios significata modos.
.[1.] circul*us*. [2.] ampulla. [3.] granu*m*.. [4.] nubecula.. [5.] spuma.
.[6.] pus. [7.] pinguedo. [8.] chim*us*. [9.] sanguis. [10.] arena. [11.] pilus.
.[12.] Squame. [13.] ffurfura. [14.] Crinoides. [15.] p*ar*tes attemose.
.[16.] Spe*r*ma. [17.] cinis. [18.] sedimen. [19.] substancia. .[20.] scintilla.
//¶\\ Spiss*us* in vrina si ci*r*cul*us* est & aquosus.
Cellula post*er*ior ffleumate pressa dolet.
//¶\\ Purpure*us* spiss*us* affligit sanguine*m* /prima\.
Leua*m* ffelle nigro pallid*us* et tenuis.
Dext*era* parte fu*er*it col*er*e fferuentis acumen.
Si tenuis fu*er*it circul*us* cit*r*in*us*. *vel*. Rube*us* atq*ue* coloris.
Insinuat sens*us* radicem mortificari.
Plu*m*be*us* & ramis hinc nocume*n*ta dari.
Deliuente p*r*ius si post rubens videatur.
Exurgat natura cerebri viroris rep*ar*at*ur*.
f. 27v Si forma*m* causon in febre virores ad/o\ptat.
ffeleus ad motu*m* frenesis su/c\ungit*ur* humor.
Si t*r*emulus fu*er*it spinalia me*m*b*ra* g*ra*uant*ur*.
Si nig*er* extiterit. *ve*l. mortificat. *ve*l. adurit.
P*r*eueniens viror *uel* liuor distinguit utru*m*q*ue*.

¶ the cerkyl is þe ouyr p*ar*t of þe vryn. and shewyth þe disposicion *and* þe greffe of þe me*m*brys of lyff as the brayn. *and* such oþ*er*. Egidi*us*. & auice*nna*.

¶ a cerkyl pure Red. *and* thicke betokenyth þ*at* the forme p*ar*t of þe hed is gr*e*uyd be blood because of ffume rysyng from þe lyu*er*. Egidi*us*.

¶ also a cerkyl whitysh watry aperyng in a vryn thick of substau*n*ce betokenyth þ*at* þe hed behynd i*n* þe Calle of mynde is g*r*evyd because of

2225 /prima\] *cancel.* proama | **2234** ad/o\ptat] *cancel.* adaptat

2216 Ipocras] *ins. by suprascr.* hypocras contentis *m.r.* | vera] *corr. by exp. and suprascr.* firma *m.r.* | **2222** scintilla] *corr. by exp.* spirit*us* apete*ns* *m.r.*
2225 /prima\] *suprascr.* prima *m.r.* | **2226** Leuam…tenuis] *corr. by exp.* //leua*m* felle nigro pallidus et tenuis\\ *m.r.* | **2232** Deliuente] *corr. by exp. and suprascr.* deliue*n*te *m.r.* | **2233** Exurgat] *corr. by exp. and subscr.* surgat *m.r.* | viroris] *corr. by exp. and subscr.* vigor *m.r.* | **2234** virores] *corr. by exp. and suprascr.* viror/i\s *m.r.*
ad/o\ptat] *suprascr.* ad/o\ptat *m.r.* | **2235** su/c\ungitur] *corr. by exp. and suprascr.* succe*n*ditur *m.r.* | **2236** spinalia] *ins. by suprascr.* id est spondila *m.r.* | **2238** uel] *corr. by exp. and suprascr.* aut *m.r.* | **2246** blood] *ext. marg.* blood

2230 Insinuat…mortificari] A change of metre to hexameters.

THE CIRCULE is thouer part of thuryn and shewith the disposition and the gref of the membres of lif as the brayn, and souch other Egid*ius*, et Auic*enna*

¶ A circule pur*e* red and thik betokneth that the forme part of the hede is greved be blode because of fume rising from the lyver, Egid*ius*.

¶ CIRCULE whitish watery appering in an vrin thik of substanc*e* betokneth that þe hede behynd in the calt of mynde is greved because of flewm*us* feume rising from the longis to that place Egid*ius*.

Cercul red lik safron tokneth the right side of thede is grevid of red coler bre*nn*y*n*g of a fume rising from the gal Egid*ius*. /

Circule pale and thyn or blac betokneth the lefte syde of the hede is grevid w*ith* melancoly of a fume rising fro the mylt Egid*ius*.

Circul that is ledish or pale tokneth

1840 the] *cancel.* p

1834 blode] *ext. marg.* ¶ Blood | **1839** flewmus] *ext. marg.* ¶ fleume | **1843** coler] *ext. marg.* ¶ Coler | **1848** melancoly] *ext. marg.* ¶ Melancoly

fflewm*us* fume rysyng from þe lu*n*g*is* to þ*a*t place. Egidi*us*.

¶ a cerkyl red lyke safferon betokenyth þe Ryȝtte syde of þe hed is g*re*uyd w*ith* red col*er* bre*n*ny*n*g of a fume rysyng from þe galle. Egidi*us*.

¶ a cerkyl pale. *and*. thy*n*ne. or black betokenyth the leffte syde of þe hed is g*re*vyd w*ith*. male*n*coly. of a ffume Rysyng from þe mylte. Egidi*us*.

¶ also a cerkyl þ*a*t is ledysh or pale betokenyth sykenes takyn of ffer*e* w*ith* ffeyntnes at þe herte. or the ffallyng. i*d est*. mortifi{ca}c*i*on of þe brayn. *and* betoken*yth* deth somtyme. Gilb*ertus*. in li*bro*. 2. ca*pitul*o. de
f. 28r dolore capitis. | w*ith* grete peyne i*n* þe back. *and* in þe Senuys. for as the brayn ffeblyth. þe senuys ffeblyn. for they haue þ*er* wexyng of þe baryn./ and yf þe ledy cerkyl turne into red it betokenyth warysshyng. *and* helthe. Egidi*us*.

¶ also. a ledy cerkyl betoken*yth* pestilence. ysaac. //¶\\ also. a cerkyl bryȝtt blew if it quake it betokenyth deth. and. a cerkyl þ*a*t q*ua*kyth betoken*yth* g*re*te i*n* þe reggebon ende. //ysaac.\\

¶ also. a cerkyl þ*a*t is grene i*n* a *con*ti*nu*al ffeu*er* as is causon þe ffeu*er* is bred p*r*incipali of coler. *and* next of blood or a ffeu*er* t*er*cian. and betokenyth g*re*te peyne in þe hed. and bre*n*ny*n*g in stomak. and if it. aper*e* in an hote accesse þan it betokenyth. a ffre*n*sy. þ*a*t comyth of col*er* ysaac.

¶ also. a black cerkyl somtyme it betokenyth a ffrensy to com. or ell*is* redy i*n* þe p*er*sone because of coler forbrent rysyng vp to þe hed befor*e*. a black cerkyl betokenyth hum*er*is be ded. *and* forbrent //¶\\ and if it be grenyssh before black. þan it betoken*yth* forbre*n*ny*n*g. //¶\\ and it be ledysh befor*e* black. þan it betokenyth veny*m*my*n*g as pestile*n*ce. &c. ysaac.

¶ also. a cerkyl thicke. and black. sig*nifica*t mortem. Egidi*us*.

//¶\\ also. a black cerkyl. thick. *and* watry. betokenyth grete hedach. grete

2252 fflewmus] *ext. marg.* fflewme | **2256** coler] *ext. marg.* Coler | **2260** malencoly] *ext. marg.* malencoli | **2281** grene] *ext. marg.* grene

siknesse takyn of fere w*ith* faintnesse at tharte the fallyng i*d est* mortification of the brayn. and betokneth deth sumtym Gilbert*us* in Li*bro* 2. ca*pitul*o de Dolore capit*is* w*ith* great payn in the bak and in the senuys, ffor as the brayn febleth the senous feblen ffor thei haue ther wexyng of the brayn ¶ And if the ledy colour turn into red it tokneth warisshing of helth Egid*ius*.

¶ Also a ledy cercul betokneth pestilens, Ysaac. Also a cercule lyght blew if it quake it tokneth deth and a Cercul that quaketh tokneth grete in the reggebone end Ysaac.

¶ Circul grene in a contynual feu*er* as is causon the feuer this feu*er* is bred principally of coler and next of blood, or a feuer tercian and tokneth grete payn in thede and bre*n*nyng in the stomoch And if it apper in a hote accesse than it tokneth a frensy that comyth of col*our* Ysaac.

¶ Also a blac cercule su*m*tym it tokneth a frensy to cu*m* or els redy in the p*er*son because of coler forbrent and ded And if it be gre*n*nysh befor blac than it tokneth forbrenny*n*g And it be ledysh before blac than it tokneth veny*mm*y*n*g as pestilenc*e* &c Ysaac

¶ Circule thik and blac sig*nifica*t mortem Egid*ius*.

¶ Circule blac thik and watery tokneth great hedach, great peyn in the forhed, and themraud*is*. and pay{n} in the chynebone ende the which cu*m*yth fro*m* the gret veyn in the forhede and so forth Egid*ius*.

1886 payn] *emend.* pay

peyne in þe for*e*hed. *and* þe Emrawdys *and* peyne in þe Chyneboon ende þe wech comyth from þe grete veyne in þe for*e*hed *and* so fforþ. Gilb*ertus*.

f. 28v Non residens ampulla tumens ventosa cohere*ns*.
Morby crudificat causam morbu*m* q*ue* p*ro*pagat.
Et nefresim gen*er*at cerebr*umque* dolore molestat.
Rugitu*m* ventris vomitu*m* facit atq*ue* dolore*m*

¶ ampulla. is a bolme. or. a burbyl. yf such burblys abyde stylle afft*er* þe vryn haue his kyndly resydence. þ*a*t is eu*er*mor*e* causyd of myxtio*un* of hum*er*is. and of ventosite enclosyd in þe body. Egidi*us*.

¶ also the burblys resydent. *and* grete. *and* bolne. *and* yf þe vryn {be} wan in colo*ur*. and it cleue hard to þe cerkyl. or to þe syde of þe vrynal. *and* wyl nat breke. þan it is. a wycked tokyn. and it betoken*yth* þ*a*t þe maledy hath takyn his dwellyng. *and* is rotyd in þe body. and yf þe burblys ben bloo. or wan. *and* grete. *and* bolne i*n* wo*m*men it betoken*yth* moch ventosyte. *and* wyckyd hum*er*is in þe mat*ri*ce. Egidi*us*.

¶ also ampulla whan it is w*ith* louhȝ colo*ur* it betokenyth þe ston in þe reynes. and Indigestion and viscouse mat*er* in the stoma k. *and* the hedach. *and* wyndy mat*er* in þe wombe as þe colyk. and if it byde styll hool afft*er* þe vryn haue his ky*n*dly restyng it betoken*yth*. harde sykenes. and long. //¶\\ and when þe wyckyd ffume. f. 29r arysyth vp in | to þe hed then þe vryn is hiy*er* //*and* a grete cerkyl.\\ in colo*ur*. afforysm*us*. 7°. *continua*. 32.

¶ also they betokenyn rawe hum*er*is. and vomytys. *and* þe ffrenesy. *and* p*er*el. ysaac.

Granula rewmatice semp*er* su*n*t nu*n*cia cause.
In circi serie si g*ra*nula fixa tenent*ur*.
In cerebro secreta latet *con*fusio morbi.
Si su/b\stent dep*re*ssa par*um* nec mota regressu*m*.
Accelerent capiti loca p*ro*xima p*er*cutit humor.

AMPULLA is a bolme or a burbyl ¶ yf f. 14v souch burbill*is* abide styl after the vryn haue his kyndly residenc*e* that is euermor caused of mixtion of humors and of ventosite enclosed in the body Egid*ius*.

¶ Also the burbils resident and great, and bolne and if thuryn be wan in colour and it cleve hard to the cerkil or to the side of the vrynal and wil not breke than it is a wiked token and it tokneth that the malady hath take his dwelling and is rottid in the body And if the burbles be blo or wan and grete and bolne in wo*m*men it tokneth ventosite and moch humeris in the matric*e* Egid*ius*.

¶ Also ampulla whan it is w*ith* lowe colour it tokneth the ston in the reynes and indigestion and viscouse matt*er* in the stomok and thedeache and wyndy matt*er* in thwombe as the colik And if it bide stil hole after thurin haue his kindly resting it tokneth hard siknesse and long And whan the wiked fume ariseth up to thede than thuryn is hy and a great cerkil in colour afforism. 7°. *content* 32.

Also thei betokyn raw humours and vomytes and frensy and perel Ysaac./

2314 haue] *cancel.* ferebro | **2319** and[2]] *rep.* and

2316 and] *corr. by exp. and suprascr.* acceler/a\nt *m.r.* | **2326** wommen] *ext. marg.* m*ulier*

2345 Granula…2346 tenentur] Note the repetition of verses 2315-2316.

P*ro*nior ad pa*r*tem fit ffluxus debiliorem.

.¶ granu*m*. *uel*. *gra*nula be litel greynes. and they {ben} as it wer*e* of chyppyng of þe spume. but it taryet leng*er*. *and* comyth fferd*er* þan doth spuma. and is somtyme i*n* þe cerkyl. somtyme vnd*er* þe cerkyl and somtyme i*n* eu*er*y region of þe vryn. Egidi*us*.

¶ and such greynes apere in þe cerkyl it betokenyth þe Rewme in þe hed. and they aper*e* in þe garlon /i*n*\ þe pipys. and they apere vnd*er* þe cerkyl. the Rewme in þe breste. Egidi*us*. //¶\\ and þe Rewme of þe sp*irit*ual me*m*bris. Gordian*us*. and somtyme it betokenyth *con*seyvyng of chyld. ysaac.

. Nubecula. a Clowde. Nebula.
Corp*or*is aerij nubecula sp*irit*ualis.
Indicat offense viciu*m* iecoris q*ue* calore*m*.

f. 29v ¶ Nubecula is a litel cloude. yf such apere i*n* þe vryn it betoken*yth* þe vice of þe sp*irit*ual me*m*bris as þe h*er*te. þe lu*n*g*is*. *and* such oþ*er*. and þ*a*t may ye knowe be the spume þ*a*t is þe scom. ffor in the vice of sp*irit*ual hete. the spume is yelwe. and in þe vice of þe sp*irit*ual me*m*bris. þe spume is ledysh. and i*n* þe vice of þe lyu*er* þe spume is redysh lyke saferon. Gordian*us*.

¶ also yf such a clowde. aper*e* dy*m*mysh. wat*r*ish. *and* blooysh hovyng above moch lyke toward a narowhweb or as it wer*e* poud*er* struwyd þ*er*y*n*ne. and it is þe sup*er*fluyte of þe. 3. digestio*u*n causyd. *and* Engendryd be onkynde hete in the lyu*er*. and in þe breste. ysaac.

¶ also it betokenyth þe ffeuer Etyk. or ellis þe body moch dissposyd þ*er*to. ysaac.

¶ also yf þe Clowde be yelwe it betoken*yth* scaldyng of þe lyu*er*. and empostyms in the lyu*er*. *and* moch Rawe mat*er*. *and* streytnes at þe brest. *and* dyst*ro*bulance of hum*er*is. *and* yf it laste long it is drede of þe hote d*r*opsy. *and* pluresis yf þe vryn be a

2361 /in\] *cancel.* þe | 2362 apere] *cancel.* in þe

2351 granum] *ext. marg.* Grana | 2375 spume] *ext. marg.* spuma

GRANU*M* uel granula be litil greynes and thei be as it war chipping of spume but it tarieth longer and cu*m*yth farther than doth spume and is su*m*tym in the cercule su*m*tym vnd*er* the cercule and su*m*tym in euery region of thurin Egid*ius*.

And souch greynes apper in the cerkil it tokneth rewme in thede and thei apper in the garlon the pipis, and thei appere vnd*er* the circul the rewme in the brest and the rewm of the sp*irit*ual me*m*bres Gordian*us*. Egid*ius* / And sumtym it tokneth conceyving of chylde Ysaac./

NUBECULA is a litil cloude Yf souch apper in thurin it tokneth the vice of the spiritual membres as tharte the lung*is* and such other And that may ye know bi the spume that is the scom ffor in the vice of sp*irit*ual hete the spume is yelow, And in the vice of sp*irit*ual membres the spume is ledish And in the vic*e* of the lyuer the spume is redish like safron Gordian*us*.

¶ Also if souch a cloude apper dy*m*mysh waterish or bloysh hoving above moch like toward a narow web, or as it war poud*er* strewed therin And it is the sup*er*fluite of the thirde digestion caused and engendred be vnkind hete in the lyuer and in the brest Ysaac.

Also tokneth the feu*er* Etik or els the body disposed moch therto Ysaac.

¶ Also if the clowd be yelow it tokneth scalding of the lyu*er* and empostyms in the liuer and moch raw matter and streitnes at the brest and disturbulans of humors And if it last long it is drede of thote dropsy ande pleuresis, Yf thurin be a pa*r*ty blew it tokneth feyntnesse at | tharte shortnese f. 15r
of breth that cu*m*yth of the lung*is* and payn in the brayn. and if it be blac it is dethe, Ysa*ac*. Gordian*us*.

¶ Also whan it is white it tokneth flewme in the pipis {than} thurin is

1935 tokneth] *cancel.* conse

. iij. causys of ffroth. because of grete mocyon of þe lu*ngis*. because of Rysi*n*g *and* bolny*n*g of þe lu*ngis*. because of ventosite aboute þe lu*ngis*.

¶ also spuma þ*a*t is blackysh is malencoly. anameli yf it com w*ith* þe colour*e* of vryn y*n*nopos. and betokenyt þe black Iawndys. and swellyng of þe galle./ and yf it be black affte*r* liuid*us*. or virid*is* it betokenyth adusty*u*n. *and* mortifycacio*u*n. Gordian*us*.

¶ also spume as it wer*e* red wyn. in vryn of Ruffe colo*ur*. it is an evyl syngne. Gordian*us*.

¶ also spume. i*n*. a wo*m*manys wat*er* betokenyth moch wynd. and peyne in
f. 31v þe sydys most in þe Ryȝht syde. | and if þe vryn be Ryȝt Cler*e*. it is peyne in þe mat*r*ice in the riȝt side. *and* þe spume be litel and thick w*ith* depe colo*ur* it is deth. Ioh*anes de sancto amando*.

betokneth moch wind and payn in the sidis most in the right side And If thurin be right clere it is payn in the matrice in the right side And the spume be litil and thik w*ith* depe colour it is deth I*ohanem*. d*e*. *sancto*. a*mando*

. Sanyes. pus. quitt*er*. att*ur*. all is on.
Vlcera vesice. sanies effusa fatet*ur*.
Aut renu*m* scabies si g*ra*uis assit odor.
Ex epatis regione finit sedime*n* saniosu*m*.
Hoc dolor. & p*ar*tis accio lesa probat.

¶ also Sanyes is eu*er*mor*e* blodysh. or red saff whan it is of þe reynes. and þan it smellyth mor*e* than whan it is of þe lyu*er*. and þ*a*t is because þe lyu*er* is hote. *and* moyste. and the Reynes is hote. *and*. drye *and* this sanies is as it wer*e* of fuske. or liuid*us* colo*ur* and is alwey vyscouse. *and* cloddy. Egidi*us*. & co*n*stan/tinus\. 7º.

SANIES also is euermore blodish or Red safe whan it is of the reynes, and than it smellith more than whan it is of the lyuer. That i{s} because the lyu*er* is hote and moist, and the reynes is hote and dry and thys Sanies is as it war of fuske or Liuidus colour and is alway viscouse and cloddy Egid*ius* co*n*stantin*us*. 4º

¶ also yf it wyl nat breke nor gladly. asondry thouh þe vryn be shake. but quave*r*yt in þe bottu*m* as it wer*e* þe white of. a raw eg. or as it wer*e* glet þ*a*t fallyth oftyntymes in hold folkk*is* vrinys and gleymowse mat*er*. þ*a*t is sanyes. and comy*n*ly it hayth a sauo*ur* þ*a*t is sowwer*e*. theo*philus*.

¶ Also if it wil not brek nor gladly asundry thow thurin be shaked but quauerith in the botom as it ware the white of a raw eg as it ware glett that fallyth often in olde folk*is* water and gleimouse mater that is sanies and co*m*me*n*ly it hath a sauour that is sour ptolom*eus*.

¶ also sanyes Comyth of. iij. placis of þe body. as of þe bladd*er*. þe Reynes. *and* þe lyu*er*. and þu mayst knowyn it.

¶ Also Sanies co*m*meth of thre plac*is* of the body, as of the reynes, the bladd*er*, and the lyuer, and thow maist know it be v. maner of wais. Be his residens, be his corporation. be sauour, be payn feling. and be

2513 Sanyes] *ext. marg.* attur | **2517** probat] *corr. by exp. and suprascr.* docet *m.r.*

2066 is] *emend.* it

be. v. man*er* of weyes. be his Resydence/ be his corp*or*aci*oun*/ be sauo*ur*/ be peyne felyng/ *and* be f. 32r worchyng | of þe secu*n*de digesti*oun*. Egidi*us*. //¶\\ and whan sanyes comyth of þe bladd*er*. as sone as þe vryn is made it drawyth down to þe grownde. //¶\\ and whan it is of þe lyu*er* it draw*yth* nat down. but it is mor*e* thicke downward in þe vryn. þan it is upward. //¶\\ and yf it com of þe reynes it goyth nat so sone down as whan it is of þe bladd*er*. //¶\\ and sanyes goyth mor*e* space w*ith* þe vryn whan it is of þe lyu*er*. than whan it is of þe Reynes. //¶\\ and mor*e* whan it is of þe Reynes. than whan it is of þe bladd*er*. Egidi*us*.

¶ also be his Encorp*or*acion w*ith* þe vryn. ffor yf it Com of þe bladd*er* it is noþyng Encorp*or*at w*ith* þe body of þe vryn. //¶\\ and it com of þe Reynes it is somwhatt corp*or*at w*ith* þe vryn. and if it com of þe lyu*er*. it is mykyl corp*or*at with þe vryn. Egidi*us*.

¶ also be his. odour*e*. for if it com of þe bladder it saferyth sor*e* //w*ith* a sowrysh tast\\ because þ*at* þe bladd*er* is cold i*n* kynde. w*ith* gr*e*te peyne. *and* pryckyng in þe shar*e*. //¶\\ and if it com of the Reynes. it stynkyth foulle. w*ith* grete peyne þ*er*. *and* syknes. //¶\\ and if it com from þe lyu*er*. it stynkyth nat but as pisse shud do. w*ith* grete peyne. *and* syknes on þe Ryht syde. and be worchyng of þe secu*n*de digesti*oun*. ffor if it be of þe bladd*er*. or of {þe} reynes. the secu*n*de digesti*oun* is not lettyd þ*er*by. and it be of þe lyu*er* þe secu*n*de digestion is hurt or fordoyn þ*er*by. Egidi*us*. Walteri*us*.

f. 32v ¶ also from þe lyu*er* comyth quytt*ur*. and þ*at* is white it hayth no sauo*ur* but litel. w*ith* ackth on þe riȝt syde. than þe lyu*er* rotyth. þe wech is causyd of bad dygesti*oun*. Egidi*us*.

¶ also douctourys seyn whan att*ur* apperyth i*n* vryn it betokenyth.

2549 sone] *cancel.* sonen | **2561** of] *rep.* of | **2572** syknes] *cancel.* þer

2543 bladder] *ext. marg.* .i. | **2545** lyuer] *ext. marg.* .2. | **2549** reynes] *ext. marg.* .3. | **2552** lyuer] *ext. marg.* .1. | **2556** Encorporacion] *ext. marg.* Corp*or*acion | **2580** quyttur] *ext. marg.* Epate

werking of the second digestion Egid*ius*. And whan Sanies co*m*myth of the bladd*er* as sone as the vrin is made it draweth down to the grownde ¶ and whan it is of the lyuer it draweth not down but it {is} more thik downwarde in thurin than it is vpwarde / And if it cu*m* of the reynes it goith not so sone down as whan it is of the bladder And sanyes goth more space w*ith* thurin whan it is of the lyuer than whan it is of the reynes, and more whan it is of the reynes than whan it is of the bladd*er* Egid*ius*.

¶ Also by his encorp*or*aci*on* w*ith* thurin for if it cu*m* of the bladd*er* it is nothing encorp*or*at w*ith* the body of thurin And it cu*m* of the reynes it is su*m*what corp*or*at And if it cu*m* of the lyuer it is mykel corp*or*at w*ith* thurin Egid*ius*.

¶ Also by his odour for if it cu*m* of the bladd*er* it sauourthe sore w*ith* a sowre taste because that the bladd*er* is colde in kind w*ith* great payn *and* priking in the share And if it cu*m* of the reynes it stynketh foul w*ith* great payn ther and siknes./ ¶ And if it cu*m* of the lyuer | it f. 16r tokneth that it stynkyth not but as pisse shuld do w*ith* great payn and siknesse on the right side and bi working of the second digestion ffor if it be of the bladd*er* or of the reynes the second digestion is not letted therby And it be of the lyuer the second digestion is hurte and fordon therby Egid*ius*. Walter*ius*.

¶ Also from the lyuer co*m*myth quytt*er* and that is white it hath no sauour but litil w*ith* ache on the right side than the lyuer rotteth which is caused of bad digestion Egid*ius*.

¶ Also doctores sayn, whan Att*er* apperith in vrin it tokneth empostymes, bocchis, bilis, bladders and scab, in on of these membres the lyuer, the back, the bladd*er* or the lung*is*. Whan it is of the lung*is* he spitteth att*er* whan it is broke w*ith* labour or w*ith* chough and than his

2096 space] *cancel.* of the l | **2101** of] *cancel.* thurin

2128 Atter] *ext. marg.* Atter

Empostyms bocchys. bolis. bladd*ers*. *and* scabbe. in oon of these me*m*bris. the lyu*er*. the back. þe bladder. or the lu*n*ggis./ whan it is of þe lu*n*gg*is* he spyttyth att*ur* wha*n* it is broke w*ith* labo*ur*. or w*ith* cough. and than his breth smellyth sor*e*. & pessi*m*a. e*st*. ypoc*ras*. 7°.

¶ and it is of þe bladd*er* þ*er* is white gr*a*uel in þe vryn *and* betoken*yth* þe me*m*b*er* is hurt. ut sup*ra*. theo*philus*.

¶ and it be in þe Reynes it hayth red sond w*ith* quytt*ur* //*in* þe vryn\\. *and* betoken*yth* gr*e*te sykenes þ*er*. & ut sup*ra*. ysaac.

¶ and yf it com of þe lyuer. it stynkyth nat nor hayth no sond in þe vryn. but it betoken*yth* st*ro*ng syknes //digestion hurt\\ w*ith* oþ*er* tokenys. afor*e*seyd. ysaac.

. tela aranee. pynguedo. vnctuosa. fatnes.
P*re*tendens olei forma resoluc*io* pinguis.
Cu*m* febre dissoluit totu*m* lu*m*bos sine febre.

¶ also vnd*er*stonde þ*a*t þ*er* be. ij. man*er* of fatnes i*n* vryn. i. is clepyd. vrina pinguis. þ*a*t is fatte vryn. anoþ*er* is clepyd. oleagena. þ*a*t is oylysh vryn. //¶\\ and thus shall ye knowe þe oon from þe oþ*er*. whan þe vryn hayþ in man*er* of a ffatnes. *and* gr*e*cynesse. above. as þu seyst on leen breues. f. 33r whan þu mayst nat se | þe fatnes but þu loke. aȝens þe sonne of þe liȝtt than it is callyd. vrina pinguis. //¶\\ and yf þe vryn haue w*ith* þe ffatnes. a man*er* of swartnes toward þe colo*ur* of oyle. þan it is callyd. vrina oleagina. as is comy*n*ly in lent ffeue*r*is. ypoc*ras*. 7°. ff. *contenta*. 33°. & ysaac.

¶ also vryn þ*a*t is oylish. *and* w*ith* hool ypostasis yf þe pacyent haue cold þ*er*w*ith*. salute*m*. sig*nifica*t. ysaac.

¶ also. an vryn þ*a*t is eu*er*y day changeabyl is. a bad tokyn. anamely in. a postym of the mydryff. ysaac. & auycen*na*. 4°.

¶ also. an vryn lyke Rust in. an agu. or

breth smellith sore et pessi*m*a est Ypoc*ras*. 7°.

¶ And it is of the bladder ther is white grauel in thurin it tokneth the membre is hurt ut sup*ra* Ptolom*eus*.

¶ And it be in the reynes it hath red sond w*ith* quytter in thurin and tokneth great siknesse ther & ut sup*ra* Ysaac.

¶ And if it cu*m* of the lyuer it stynketh not nor hath no sond in thurin but it tokneth strong siknesse, Indigestion hurt w*ith* other tokyns aforeseyd, Ysaac.

ALSO vnderstond that ther be ij maner of ffatnesse In thurin oon is cleped vrina pinguis. that is fat vrin / Another is cleped oleagena and that is oilysh vrin And thus shal ye know thoon fro*m* thother whan thurin hathe in maner of a fatnesse and greycenes above as thow seist on leen brewes whan thow maist not se /þe\ fatnesse but thow loke ayenst the sun or the liȝght than it is called vrina pi*n*guis And if thurin haue w*ith* the fatnesse a maner of swartnesse toward the colour of oyl than it is called vrina oleagina as is como*n*ly in lent feueres, Ypoc*ras* 7°. Ysaac.

¶ Also vrin that is oylish and w*ith* hole yposta*sis* if the pacient haue cold therw*ith* salut*em* sig*nifica*t Ysaac.

¶ An vrin that is euery day changeable is a bad token and namely in a postym of the mydrif Ysaac Auic*enna* 4°

¶ Also an vrin like rust in an agu, or moch dym tokneth that the spasme shal cum Egid*ius*.

¶ Also su*m*tym fatnesse comyth from

2590 lunggis/] *ext. marg.* pulmo*n*is | **2595** bladder] *ext. marg.* vesice | **2608** Pretendens] *ext. marg.* *versus* | **2616** ffatnes] *ext. marg.* ffatnes

2158 above] *emend.* asbove | **2159** maist] *cancel.* se

moch dym betoken*yth* þ*a*t þe spasme shall com. Egidi*us*.

¶ also somtyme. ffattnes comyth from all the body. and þ*a*t is if þe body be ffeu*erus*. //¶\\ and somtyme it comyth from þe Reynes. than þe body is w*ith* out ffeu*er*. Egidi*us*. & ysaac.

¶ and if þe vryn haue moch ffatte it betokenyth þe ffeu*er* is hote. *and* drye. and it betoken*yth* he is wastyng. *and con*sumy*ng* of kynde.

//¶\\ and oþ*er*while it betokenyth a lent ffeu*er*. w*ith* febylnesse of þe reynes. for it comyth from þe reynes. and þe vryn. *and* þe fatnes is moch in qu*an*tyte. //Egidi*us*\\

¶ and if fatnes aper*e* in vryn w*ith* a
f. 33v *con*tinual | feu*er* it betokenyth.
*con*sumyng. *and* dryyng of all þe body w*ith* gr*e*te peyne. *and* hete at þe h*er*te. anamely if þe vryn be crudy. ysaac.

//¶\\ and if it com from all þe body it betokenyth a feu*er* Etyk. þan þe ffattnes is lesse in qu*an*tyte. þen whan it comyth from þe Reynes. auer*o*iȝ. 4º.

¶ also it is to be vnd*er*stonde. þ*a*t þ*er* be. iij. dyu*er*se vryns of Etyk. the firste spice of þe etyk is droppys of oyle./ the secu*n*de is lyke. a Cobweb./ the thryde is lyke oyle. for if it wer*e* shedd on. a stoon it wyll be lyke oyle. *and* eue*r*mor*e* it betokenyth wastyng of kynde. *and* it is vncurabyl. auycen*na*. 4º. aff*orismus*. 2 º.

¶ and if oyly vryn cu*m* in þe begy*n*ny*ng* of. a syknes w*ith* oþ*er* euyl signes. morte*m* sig*nifica*t. auycen*na*. 4º.

¶ also if fattnes aper*e* w*ith* an accesse it betokenyth wastyng of gr*e*ce. aboute þe nerys. auycen*na*.

¶ and þe vryn be moch in qu*an*tyte. *and* thenne thanne þe ffatnes shewyth soon and it /be\ thenne. *and* lytel in qu*an*tyte. it betokenyth. a ffeu*er* Etyk. and þe vryn muste stonde long or þe ffatnes shewe. auycen*na*.

2661 iij] *cancel.* maner of dy | **2664** were] *cancel.* lyke | **2678** lytel] *cancel.* ke MS ly~~ke~~tel

2662 firste] *ext. marg.* .i. | **2663** secunde] *ext. marg.* .2. | **2664** thryde] *ext. marg.* .3. | **2679** Etyk] ext. marg. Raw humo*ur*

al the body, and that is if the body be feu*er*ys, and su*m*tym it co*m*myth fro*m* the reynes than the body is without feu*er* Egid*ius*. Ysaac

¶ And if thurin haue moch fat it tokneth the feuer is hote and dry. and it tokneth he is co*n*sumyng and wasting of kinde

¶ And otherwhilis it tokneth a lent feuer w*ith* feblenes of the reynes, ffor
it cu*m*yth from the reynes and thuryn | f. 16v
and the fatnesse is moch in quantite Egid*ius*.

¶ And if fatnesse apper in vrin w*ith* a co*n*tynual feuer it tokneth co*n*sumyng and dryyng of al the body w*ith* great payn and hete at tharte, and namely if thurin be crudy Ysaac

¶ And if it cu*m* fro*m* al the body it tokneth a feuer Etik than the fatnesse is Lesse in quantite than whan it cu*m*yth from the reynes Au*er*oiȝ 4º

¶ it is to be vnderstonde also, that ther be iij dyuerse vrines of the Etik The furst spice of Etik is droppis of oile ¶ The second is like a cobweb ¶ The thurd is like oyl for if it wer shed on a ston it wil be like oyl and euermore it tokneth wasting of kinde and it is vncurable auic*enna*. 4º. aff*orism* 2º

¶ And if oily vryn cu*m* in the begynny*ng* of a siknes w*ith* other evyl signes morte*m* sig*nifica*t. auic*enna* 4º.

¶ Also if fatnes appere w*ith* an axes it tokneth wasting of grese abowt the nerys Auic*enna*.

¶ And thurin be moch in qua*n*tite and thyn then the fatnesse shewyth sone, and it be thyn and litil in quantite it tokneth a feuer Etik / And thuryn must stond lo*ng* or the fatnesse shewe./ Auicen*na*.

2177 that] *cancel.* body | **2179** body] *cancel.* cu*m*yth

¶ also blood. somtyme it Comyth from þe lyuer. *and* somtyme from þe bladd*er*. and somtyme from the Reynes. *and* somtyme from a veyne þ*at* is rupt. as kylis throuh þe wech brekyng comyth þe Emrawdys. and from ech place of all these þ*at* þe blod comyth from. it is vnd*er*stonde be certeyn signys. Gordian*us*.

¶ and if þe bloo be fful of bolmys. *and* stondyng in þe botu*m*. *and* lytel. is p*er*lous. and somdel sty*n*kyng w*ith* peyne in þe shar*e*. *and* p*ri*ckyng þ*er*. and in þe ȝerdys ende and in þe fu*n*dmentte. than ito comyth from the bladd*er*. þan if it {be} mykel it is vncurabyl. Gordian*us*.

¶ and if it com of þe Reynes. it is pur*e*. *and* lytel *and* somwhat myxtt w*ith* þe vryn. and þe vryn wyll stynke. *and* signyfieþ þe ston. and grete sykenes. *and* peyne in þe back. ypoc*ras*.

¶ and if a man pisse blood. hesily. moch. *and* pure. w*ith*out cause of outward hurt it betokenyth brekyng of. a veyne in þe back. ypoc*ras*. 4°. aff*orismus*. *con*tinuo. 78°.

¶ and if it com from þe lyu*er*. it is ffayr. and clere *and* stynkyth nat w*ith* g*re*te peyne. *and* dyssese on þe ryȝht syde. betokenyth. a veyne broken. i*n* þe lyu*er* wyth oþ*er* dyssesys. *and* syknes þ*er*. Egidi*us*.

f. 35v ¶ also yf it {be} litel. *and* thycke. hauy*ng*. a st*r*ong sauou*r* and it is gobett*is* in þe botu*m* of þe vryn. than it betokenyth it comyth from þe bladd*er*. ypoc*ras*. 4°.

¶ also if blood. aper*e* long tyme in vryn. *and* moch i*n* qu*an*tyte. malu*m* sig*nifica*t. Gordian*us*.

¶ also blood in vryn as it wer*e* cloutty fflesh. *and* derk aboue. malu*m* sig*nifica*t. auycen*na*. 3°.

and he pysse blood sharpe. *and* pure //. w*ith*. a. sharpe ffeu*er*.\\ morte*m* sig*nifica*t. avycen*na*. 4°. and yf þe blood be cloddyd in a sharpe ffeu*er*. malu*m*. sig*nifica*t. auycen*na*.

2775 kylis] *cancel* kyklis | **2784** ȝerdys] *cancel*. ȝerdyd | **2792** back] *cancel*. yp

2780 bolmys] *ext. marg*. vesice | **2788** Reynes] *ext. marg*. Renes | **2799** lyuer] *ext. marg*. Epate

BLOODE also sumtym it co*m*myth from the lyuer and sumtym fro*m* the bladder, and sumtym from the reynes, and sumtym from the veyn that is rupte as kilys thorow the which breking co*m*myth themraud*is*, and from eche place of al these that the bloode co*m*myth from it is vnderstonde be certayn signis Gordian*us*

¶ And if the blo be ful of bolmys and standing in the botom and litil is p*er*lous and sumdele stinking w*ith* payn in the share and priking ther and in the yard*is* yende and in the fundament than it comyth from the bladder than if it be mykil it is vncurable, Gordianus

¶ And if it cum of the reynes it is pure and litil and sumtym myxt w*ith* thurin and thuryn wil stynk and signifieth the ston, and great siknes, and payn in the bac Ypoc*ras*

¶ And if a man pysse bloode esyli moch and pure w*ith*out cause of owtwarde hurte it tokneth breking of a veyn in the bac Ypoc*ras*

¶ And if it cum from the lyuer it is fair. and clere and stynketh not w*ith* great payn and disese in thryght syde tokneth a veyn broke in the lyuer w*ith* other diseses and siknesse ther, Egid*ius*

¶ Also if it be thik and litil hauyng a stronge sauoure and it is gobettis in the botom of thuryn than it tokneth it cometh from the bladder. Ypoc*ras* 4°.

¶ Also if blode appere longe tym in thuryn and moch in quantite malum significat, Gordianus

¶ Also bloode in vryn as it were clouty flesh and derke aboue malum sig*nifica*t Auicen*na*. 3°.

¶ And he pisse blood sharp and clere pure w*ith* a sharp feuer mortem significat. auicen*na* 4°. And if the blood be cloddede in a sharp feuer malu*m* sig*nifica*t auicen*na*

¶ And if it breke owt so because of a feuer and of great hete, and if the

2338 feuer] *cancel*. mortem

//¶\\ and if it breke out so because of a feu*er* *and* of grete hete. *and* if þe blood be medlyd w*ith* sedymen as it wer*e* curdyd it betokenyth hurtt of. a. veyn. or of. a postym in þe wey of þe vryn. auer*o*iȝ. 4°.

¶ also if it be spotty. as bloo. *and* Red then þe peyne is. i*n* þe reynes. in þe shar*e*. and in þe yerde. auycen*na*.

¶ and if it be cler*e*. *and* blak. þe peyne is in þe back. þe bladd*er*. and in þe shar*e*. auycen*na*.

bloode be medled w*ith* sedimen as it ware curdyd it tokneth hurt of a vayn or a postym in the way of the vryn auer*o*iȝ 4°.

¶ Also if it be spotty as bloo or red than the peyn is in the reynes and the share and in the ȝerde Auic*enna* f. 17v

¶ And if it be clere and blac the payn is in the bac in the bladder and in the share./ auic*enna*./

. lapidem. grauel. arena.
Renu*m* vesice lapidem testant*ur* arene.
Renu*m* si rubee. Vesice si magis albe.
Emula co*n*tenti si/c\ forma suo retinenti.

¶ arena is gr*a*uel somtyme it comyth from þe Reynes. and somtyme from þe. bladd*er*. auycen*na*. pr*imo*.

¶ and if it be red gr*a*uel it comyth from þe Reynes. *and* betokenyth þe f. 36r ston þ*er*. and if it be white. | it comyth from þe bladd*er*. *and* betokenyth þe ston þ*er*. and if it be black. and hard. *and* grett it betoken*y*t*h* of þe baldd*er* also. co*n*stantyn*us*. auer*o*iȝ. 4°.

¶ and if þe ston be nesh. *and* red it betokenyth brent blod in þe bladd*er*. or in þe lyu*er*. ysaac.

¶ and if it be in þe Reynes þe pacyent hayþ gr*e*te peyne *and* acthe þ*er*. *and* in þe haunch. ysaac.

¶ and if it be in þe bladd*er*. he ffelyth peyne in þe yerdys ende. *and* in þe flanke. ysaac.

¶ and if it be black. it comyth of malencoly. *and* then it is vncurabyl. saff oonly be cuttyng. ysaac.

¶ also þu shalt nat knowe gr*a*uel only be þe colo*ur*. wher*e* it is bred be ffelyng. *and* such oþ*er* tokenys. *and* somtyme it is red whan it /is\ nat þe ston. but somtyme it betokenyth hum*er*is forbrent in þe veynes þo {þ*at*} be nat hard in þe hand as gr*a*uel þ*at* is bred in þe reynes and it betokenyth þe artetyca passion. or þe ffeu*er* quarteyn. *and* þo be yelwe. i*d* *est*. col*er*. //¶\\ and if þey be. liuid*us*. or. black. i*d* *est*. Malencoly. it is

ARENA is grauel, Sumtym it cu*m*yth from the reynes and sumtym from the bladd*er* Auic*enna* pr*im*o.

¶ And if it be red grauel it co*m*myth from the reynes and tokneth the ston there ¶ and if it be white it co*m*meth from the bladder and tokneth the ston ther ¶ And if it be blac and harde and grete it tokneth of the bladd*er* also Co*n*sta*n*tinus, auer*o*iȝ 4°.

¶ And if the ston be nesh and red it tokneth brent bloode in the bladder, or in the lyuer Ysaac.

¶ And if it be in the reynes the pacient hath great payn and ache ther, and in the hanche Ysaac

¶ And if it be in the bladder he hath payn in the yard*is* yende and in the flanc./ Ysaac

¶ And if it be blac it co*m*meth of melancoly and then it is vncurable saue oonly be cutting Ysaac./

¶ Also thow shal not know grauel oonly be the colour where it is bredde be felyng and souch other tokyns, and sumtym it is red whan it is not the ston but sumtym it tokneth humors forbrent in the veynes tho that be not hard in the hande as grauel that is bred in the reynes, and it tokneth þe artetyca passio*n* or the feuer quarte*in* and þo be yelow i*d* *est* coler and if

2860 is] *cancel.* brent

2374 Ysaac/] *oblit.* And if it be in the reynes the pacient hath great payn | **2380** not] *cancel.* be

wickyd. *and* deþ. //¶\\ and whan it aperyth louh in þe botum of þe vryn. Red as it were Ruffe. *and* smal as it were asshys. or dust. it betokenyth scyatica passio. or nefresy. or scabbe. or saltt flewm. or þe. Etyk. or þe tysyk. or clensyng of þe splen. or of þe lyu*er*. or þe. dropsye. and specialy. þe cold d*ro*psye. s*ecundu*m. Iohanem. de. s*anct*o amando. & galyen. & Egidi*us*.

¶ and somtyme it betokenyth. a
f. 36v sympyl t*er*cian | or a dowbyl t*er*cian. Egidi*us*.

¶ Nothyng wyll brede þe ston su*nner* þan wyll drynkyng moch of wat*er*. for it causyth moyst hum*er*is. *and* gross. *and* viscouse.

. Pilis. heir.
fforma pilo similis. *ve*l. erit decisio carnis.
Aut p*ars* humoris lima siccata caloris.
Inde p*ro*bes Ren*um*. *ve*l. toci*us* nocument*um*.

¶ Pilus is an heir*e*. yf heer*e* aper*e* in vryn it comyth of hum*er*is. or of þe flesh. and betokenyth drynes of þe reynes. yf þe syke haue no ffeu*er*. //¶\\ and yf he haue no feu*er* it betokenyth drynes of all þe body. Gordian*us*. 76.

¶ also such heer*e* betokenyth syknes. *and* ach in the lendys throuht excesse of vnkynde hete wastyng þe substau*n*ce in þe Reynes./ or ell*is* þe pacyent hayth vsyd to moch wo*m*men. and so dyst*ro*yd hymselffe throuh such doyng. Gordian*us*. Egidi*us*.

¶ also it betokenyth grete thoutt. *and* viscou*s* hum*er*is in þe body. Gordian*us*. *and* sp/e\cial. i*n* þe holounesse of þe back.

¶ also if they shew them evyn long. w*ith* an accesse be fflux if they aper*e*. then it is deth. Egidi*us*.

¶ and they aper*e* w*ith*. a louh vryn it betokenyth wastyng. *and* dryyng of Reynes. and in hyȝe vryn wastyng of þe. 4. hum*er*is. Egidi*us*.

//¶\\ and they be red they com of blood. yf {they} be white they com of

thei be Liuid*us* or blac. i*d est* melancoly it is wiked and deth. ¶ And whan it aperith low in the botom of thuryn red as it were Rufe and smal as it were asshis or duste it tokneth sciatica passio, or nefresi, or scab. or salt flewm or the Etyk or the tisyk or clensing of the splen / or of the lyuer or the dropsy and specially the cold dropsi Io*hanem*. d*e*. s*ancto*. a*mando*. Egidius

¶ And sumtym it tokneth a simple tercian, or a dowble tercian Egid*ius*./

¶ Nothing wil brede the ston soner than will drynking moch of water ¶ ffor it cawseth moist humoures and grose, and Viscouse.

PILUS is an here. yf here appere in vrin it cometh of humours, or of the flesh, and tokneth dryenes {y}f the reynes of the seke haue no feuer it betokneth drynes of al the body Gordian*us*. 7

¶ Also such here tokneth siknes, and ache in the lend*is* thorow excesse of vnkind hete wasting the substans in the reynes, or els the pacient hath vsed to moch wo*m*men, and so destroyed hymself thorow souch doyng. Gordian*us*. Egid*ius*.

¶ Also it tokneth great thowght and viscous humoures in the body Gordian*us*, and speciali in holownesse of the bac

¶ Also if they shew themself evyn long w*ith* an axes be flux if they apere then it is deth Egid*ius*./

¶ And thei apper with a low vrin | it f. 18r
tokneth wasting and driyng of the reynes ¶ And in the hye vryn wasting of the 4 humors Egid*ius*.

¶ And they be red they cu*m* of bloode / yf thei be white they cu*m* of flewme

2398 ston] *cancel.* sonder | **2403** here[2]] *cancel.* of | **2404** cometh] *cancel.* or | **2405** yf] *emend.* of | **2424** of] *rep.* of

2877 þe] *cancel.* st

f. 37r fflewm. yf they be yelwe. they com | of col*er*. yf they com of Malencoly //black\\. Gordian*us*.

¶ also for to knowe them bett*er*. ffele hem in þi ffyngrys sofftly. *and* if þu ffele in man*er* of sadnes as it wer*e* fflesh. than it is of þe fflesh. *and* if it be cont*ra*ry it is of oþ*er* hum*er*is. Gordian*us*.

Scalis. Squames.
P*er* squanus tenues. aut furfura Iu*n*cta notat*ur*.
Vesice scabies aut si febris comitatur.
Loci*us* fluit integ*ri*tas corpus tenuatur.

¶ Squame is lesse. *and* thy*n*ner than is ffurfura and betokenyth þe firste spice of þe etyk. *and* comyth moste of þe sp*iti*tual*is*. and than it is vpward in þe vryn. //¶\\ and if it be louh in þe vryn thanne it comyth of þe bladd*er*. and if it be ouer all i*n* þe vryn. thanne it com*yth* of all p*ar*tiys of þe body. Egidi*us*.

¶ and. ypoc*ras*. *and* galyen seyn þ*at* squame comyn of me*m*brys þ*at* ben webby. as veynes arteries *and* senuys and such*e* oþ*er*. this squames is like scalys of ffysh. and yf such aper*e* w*ith*out feu*er* it comyth of þe bladd*er*. oftyn dissevyng þe leche demyng þe ston i*n* þe bladd*er*. whan it is scabbe. Egidi*us*.

¶ and if it be white w*ith*. a ffeu*er*. it betokenth þ*at* all þe body waxyth lene. *and* dryeth up. & pessi*ma*. e*st*. analy if they be white. soffte. *and* smoth. *et* peior e*st*. Egidi*us*.

¶ also squames. or pentoloyde. þe wech ar all of on signifycacion. and if
f. 37v they be brode they be | token a ffeu*er* etyck meltyng. *and* wastyng þe body. w*ith* all*e* oþ*er* sig*n*is of furfura. þe wech ffolwyth. Gilbert*us*.

. ffurfurea. ffarencas. brenn.

¶ and bren aper*e* in vryn it betokenyth syknes of þe bladd*er*. as scabbis. þ*at* comyn of vnkynde hete. or ell*is* of a ffeu*er* etyk. *and* if it be w*ith* an excesse it betokenyth þe fyrste spice

Yf they be yelow they cu*m* of Coler. if thei be bloo they cu*m* of melancoli Gord*ianus*.

¶ Also for to know them better, fele the*m* in thi fingers softly and if thow fele in maner of sadnes as it war fleshe than it is of the flesh. and if it be contrary it is of thum*ers* Gord*ianus*.

SQUAME is les and thy*n*ner than is furfura and tokneth the first spice of thetyk and co*m*myth most of the sp*irit*uall*is* and than it is vpward in thuryn, and if it be low in thurin then it co*m*meth from the bladder. and if it be ouer al in thuryn than it co*m*meth of al the p*ar*ties of the body Egid*ius*./

¶ And ypoc*ras* and galen seyn that squame co*m*myth of membres that be webby as veynes arteries and senuous and souch other, this squames is like scal*is* of fish, and if souch apper w*ith*out feuer it tokneth of the bladd*er* often deseyuyng the leche demyng the ston in the bladd*er* whan it is the scab. Egid*ius*

¶ And if it be white w*ith* a feuer it tokneth that al the body waxeth lene, and drieth up et pessima est, and namely if they be white, softe, and smoth et peior est. Egid*ius*

¶ Also squames, or petoloide, the which ar al of on signification, and if thei be brode thei betoken a feu*er* Etik melting and wasting the body w*ith* al other signes of furfura the which foloweth Gilbert*us*.

¶ ffurfura. farencas bren*e*./

ANDE BREN aper in vrin it tokneth siknes of the bladd*er*, as scabbes that cu*m* of an vnkind hete. or els of a feuer etik / ¶ And if it be w*ith* an axes it tokneth the first spic*e* of thetyk / so

2929 squanus] *corr. by exp. and suprascr.* squan/a\s *m.r.* | **2930** aut] *corr. by exp. and suprascr.* vel *m.r.* | **2931** fluit] *ins. by suprascr.* petit *m.r.*

2434 of] *cancel.* sand | **2448** be] *cancel.* welly

hondys. Sciatica *in* þe hau*n*che. Gutta rosacea *in* þe face. artetica. *in* þe loyntt*is*.

¶ What goutte so eu*er* it be þe vryn is euyrmor*e* bloo. abovyn. þ*at* is derk. *and* dym. and somtyme þe goutte is in þe riȝt halffe. *and* somtyme in þe leffte syde. and somtyme in bothe but in þe leffte syde is eu*er*more p*er*el. Egidi*us*.

¶ and yf þe motis aper*e* in {þe} ou*er* p*ar*t of þe vryn than they betoken þe rematyk goutte in the breste. and if they aper*e* in þe mydel Regioun it betoken*yth* þe rewmatyk goutte in þe stomak. *and* in þe lyu*er*./ and if they aper*e* in þe g*ro*unde of þe vryn it betokenyth þe goutte in þe reynes./ and if it stonde stylle shakyng it betokenyth þe rennyng goutte. Egidi*us*.

¶ and it aper*e* swart and *tro*bly in a wo*m*manys vryn it betokenyth Rysy*ng*
f. 39v of her*e* | matr*i*ce //¶\\ and if it falle down to þe botom of þe vrynal lu*m*ppy as it wer*e* whete flour*e* it betokenyth w*ith*holdyng of hyr*e* fflourys. Egidi*us*.

¶ also yf it aper*e* in þe vryn smal and black. //¶\\ and in þe botom it betoken*yth* peyne in þe Ryȝtt syde. þe wech is of a postym. *id est*. p*er*ilpleumo*n*ia. &. plueresis. Gilb*er*t*us*.

¶ this *con*tentt attomys betoken*yth* p*ri*ncipaly. iij. thyng*is*. the goutt*is*. sykenes of þe matrice or Concepcio*u*n. Egidi*us*. & Gordian*us*.

¶ also for to knowyn whan. a wo*m*man is conseyvyd. drawyng. *and* suckyng on þe ma*n*nys yerde. nor she lustyth nat to company wyth ma*n*. nor her*e* me*m*b*er* wosyth nat nor yevyth so mykel moystour*e* outward as it dede beffor*e*. and whan she is conceyvyd hir*e* fflourys ar*e* stoppyd. she hayþ dyu*er*se appetit*is* to dyu*er*s met*is* and drynk*is*. *and* moch dysposyd to p*ar*brakyng bycause of walmyng. *and* rysyng up to þe stomak by cause hir*e* fflour*is* ben Ryȝt vnstabyl tyl þe thryd month or þe.

su*m*tym in both*e* but in the lefte side is euermore perel Egidi*us*.

¶ And if the mot*is* aper in thouer p*ar*te of thuryn the{i} tokyng the reumatik gout in the brest ¶ And if thei aper in the medil region it tokneth the reumatik gout in the stomoc / and in the lyuer, And if the{y} aper in the ground of thurin it tokneth the gout in the reynes ¶ And if it stond stil shaking it tokneth the re*n*nyng gout Egid*ius*.

¶ And it aper swart and trobly in a | f. 19r
wommans vrin it tokneth rising of her matrice ¶ And if it fal down lumpy, as it were whete flour, it tokneth w*ith*holding of her flour*is* Egid*ius*

¶ Also if it aper smal and blac in the botom it tokneth payn in the right side the which is of an Empostym *id est* p*er*ipleumonia vel pleure*sis* Gilbert*us*

¶ This content Athom*us* tokneth iij thing*is* the gout siknesse of the matrice Egid*ius* Gordian*us*.

¶ Also for to know {whan a womman} is co*n*ceyued w*ith* drawing and sucking of the ma*n*nys yarde, not she lestith to co*m*pany w*ith* man, nor her membre hosith not nor gef nat so moch moister outwarde as it dyd before. and whan she is co*n*ceyued her floures is stopped she hath dyuerse appetit*is* to metys and drynk*is*, and moch disposed to p*ar*brake because of walmyng and rising up to the stomok because her flour*is* be right vnstable tyl the thirde month or the fourth. than her pappis swel and wex greit. and the attomys apper in vrin of a woman so that thei be thik downwarde like water that Amido*n* war wasshyn in and sone {after} thei gathern and clodyn together it tokneth that she is co*n*ceyued

¶ And (as auic*enna* sayth) if ther aper in thuryn a thyn body moch toward raw silke, and than thattomes be red or rody or smale the colour of the pappis changing ande swelling. and if the ey wex red and sumwhat ledy abowte in her face, nek, and hand*is*

3076 þe[1]] *cancel.* mydel reg

3099 conseyvyd] *ext. marg. conce*pcio | **3100** yerde] *int. marg.* man

2560 if] *cancel.* s

forthe./ þan hir*e* pappis sw/e\ll *and* wexyn g*re*te/ and if attomys aper*e* in vryn of a wo*m*man so þ*at* þey be f. 40r thycke anamely down | ward lyke wat*er* þ*at* amydown whe wasshyn y*n*ne and soon aft*er* þey gad*er*en. *and* Cloddyn toged*er* it betokenyth þ*at* she is co*n*seyuyd.

and as auicen*na* seyth yf þ*er* aper*e* in þe vryn a thy*n*ne body white moch toward raw sylke and than þo attomys be red or rody *and* smale þe colo*ur* of þe pappys choyngyn. *and* swellyn. *and* ytchyn þe eyen wexyn rede. *and* somwhatt ledy abowtt. and in hir*e* fface. necke. *and* handys wexyn somtyme spott*is*. *and* ffraklys. and if hir*e* fface be bryȝtt. and hir*e* ly*m*mys lyȝtsom. *and* hir*e* wombe rownde. hir*e* mylke thicke it betokenyth þ*at* she is conseyvyd w*ith* a man chy{l}de *and* if it be *contra*ry it is a wo*m*man chylde.

¶ also yf þ*er* be ffowndyn in þe vryn. iij greynes nat sondryth. sig*nifica*t co*n*cepci*on* auycen*na*.

¶ also the. i. or þe. 2. or þe. 3. month þe vryn shall haue smale clowdys w*ith*y*n*ne. w*ith* a white grow*n*de and þe vryn shal be riȝt cler*e* *and* shy*n*ny*n*g. and þey þ*at* be. 4. monthys goyn þ*er* vryn shal be cler*e* red. *and* þe g*ro*wnde white shy*n*ny*n*g. auycen*na*.

sumtyme wex spottis and frackils, and if her face be bright, et her ly*m*mes litsum, and her wombe rownd her mylk thik it tokneth she is co*n*ceyued w*ith* a man child

¶ Also if ther be fownd in thuryn thre greynes sig*nifica*t co*n*ceptione*m*

¶ Also the first, the second or the third monthe thuryn hath smale clowd*is* within w*ith* a white grownde and thurin shal be right clere and shyni*n*g and þei þ*at* be 4 monthis going ther vrin shal be clere red, and the grownde white shyni*n*g Auic*enna*./

. Cineris. or. asshys.
Sub fforma cin*er*is corpuscula p*re*ssa deorsu*m*.
Infima me*mbra* nota*n*t morbi lang\u/ore g*ra*uari.
f. 40v Exat*r*icis emorroidis splenis q*ue* tunore.
Sepius aparent. *ve*l. qua*n*do menst*ru*is humor.
Temp*or*ib*us* certis sua respiracula nescit.

¶ also Cin*er*is ben asshys yf þey aper*e* in þe vryn //and p*r*incipally it betoken*yth* wasty*n*g of the lu*n*gg*is*. *and* consu*m*pci*o*n of þe body.\\ it betokenyth syknes. *and* dissesys benethforth as fic*us*. or þe emrawdys. and þe tetis or bigg*us* of þe emrawdys to swoln. Egidi*us*.

¶ also swellyng of þe mylte. and spottyng of wo*m*men fflux oftyntymes Gordian*us*.

Also cineres. be ashis and principalli tokneth wasting of the lung*is* and co*n*su*m*ption of the body. it tokneth siknes and diseses benethfor as or themraud*is* and the tetis of the bigg*is* of themraud*is* be swolen Egid*ius*.

Or of swelling of the mylte spotting of wome*n* flux oftentymes Gord*ianus*.

¶ Also in wome*n* it tokneth siknes of her matric*e* thorow retention of

---

3121 þe] *cancel.* aper*e* | **3156** emrawdys] *cancel.* em~~ra~~rawdys

3112 þan] *ext. marg.* Re*w*le | **3114** vryn] *ext. marg.* vryn

2622 the[2]] *cancel.* lung*es* | **2625** of[3]] *cancel.* wo*m*man

¶ also in wo*m*men it betoken*yth* sykenes {of} hire mat*ri*ce through rete*n*cion of malencoly humer*is*. ¶ and if asshys aper*e*. *and* þe vryn be lowh of colo*ur*. wi*th* black *and* bloo Resolucions beyng in þe botom then it betokenyth þe Emrawdys. or att*ri*ces or Condolomata. &. ficus. ysaac.

¶ and if þe *con*tentis be black. or bloo. or pu*r*pyl wi*th* a lowh colo*ur* it betokenyth stoppyng of þe ffloury

//¶\\ asshys in vryn att*ery* betoken*yth* þe emrawdys. yf þe colo*ur* be liuyde. ysaac.

¶ and wi*th* g*re*nys or yerdys it betokenyth swellyng of þe splen. *and* al these com of malencoly. ysaac.

melancoly humo*urs* ¶ And if ashes aper in vrin that is of low /of\ colour wi*th* blac and blo resolutions being in the botom it tokneth themraud*is*, or Att*ri*ces / or Condolomata vel ficus Ysaac.

¶ And if the contentis be blac or blo or purpil wi*th* a low colour it tokneth stopping of the flourys.

Asshis in thuryn Attery tokneth f. 19v
themraud*is* if the colour be liuide Ysaac

¶ And wi*th* greynes, or yerd*is* it tokneth swelling of the splen ¶ And al these comyth of melancoly Ysaac./

. Sparma. seed. or kynde.
Spermaticis insc*ri*pta notis vrina fatet*ur*.
Illecebres Chitus genitalia me*m*b*ra* g*ra*uari.
ffermen*t*o veneris. ludibria vana soporis.
f. 41r Sine go norrea*m*. *v*el me*m*bri vim resoluta*m*.

¶ Sparma is a ma*n*nys or. a wo*m*manys seed or kynde. þe wech hath his ffirste grownde in þe brayn and so goyth forth to þe gen*er*ati*ui*s. ysaac.

¶ and sp*ar*me aper*e* in vryn it betokenyth. moch hawntyng. or Company wi*th* wo*m*men befor*e*. or polucyon in sleple. or grete dyssyr*e* to wo*m*men. or palsy of ma*n*nys gen*er*ati*ui*s. þ*a*t is þe vessel þ*a*t shuld kepe þe sed. or be gomorrea passion that is onwyhful shedyng of seed. or for ffebylte þ*a*t he may nat hold it but slepyng or wakyng it passyth awey. throuh þe wech cause bothe men and wo*m*men die oftyntymes. ysaac.

¶ also sp*ar*ma C*ri*solomeris. yf þey aper*e* flety*n*g above in þe vryn and þe vryn be Raw in colo*ur* it betoken*yth* passyng of kynde //wi*th*out lykyng.\\ and if they aper*e* in hey colo*ur*d vryn. þen it betokenyth þ*a*t it was made post s*u*bpositu*m*. ysaac.

¶ also whan sp*ar*me aperyth lyke tosyd woll it betokenyth vanyteis in slepe. ysaac.

¶ also if it aper*e* i*n* g*re*te qua*n*tyte wi*th* entens and thycke vryn *and* lowh

SPERMA is a ma*n*nys or a womans sede, or kinde the which is first grownyd in the brayn and so goth forth to the generatyuys Ysaac./

¶ And sp*er*me in vrin appere it tokneth moch hawnting or co*m*pany of women befor or polution in slepe, or great desir to wo*m*men, or palsy of memb*ry*s generati*ui*s that is the vessel that shuld kepe the sede, or be gomorai passion, that is, an onwilful sheding of sede, or for febelte that he may nat hold it, but sleping or waking it passith away fro*m* hym, thorow thwich cause both men and women dey oftentymes Ysaac.

¶ Also sp*er*ma cu*m* solomeris if thei apper fleting above in thuryn, and thuryn be raw in colour it tokneth passing of kind wi*th*out likinge And if the{i} aper in hie coloured vrin than it tokneth it was made post subpositu*m* Ysaac

¶ Also whan sp*er*me appereth like tosed woll it tokneth vanyteis in slepe Ysaac /

// Also if it aper wi*th* great quantite wi*th* ententic*e* and thik vrin and lowgh nat fully in the botom it tokneth rancor of moch blood Gomorea is

3180 fatetur] *ins. by suprascr.* id *est* signat *m.r.* | **3181** Chitus] *corr. by exp. and suprascr.* coitus *m.r.*

nat ffully in þe botom it betokenyth gomor*e* of moch blood. gomorrea is pouryng out of sed of man. or wo*m*man wylfully aȝens kynde. ysaac.

f. 41v ¶ also if it aper*e* wan. *and* w*ith* remyshnes. *and* thy*n*ne it betoken*yth* gomor*e* of ffebylnes. ysaac.

¶ also asshis in vryn betokenyth dyssesis of þe splen. of þe mat*ri*ce. of þe emrawdys. ye shall nat dysserne well oon from ano*þer* be colo*ur*. for whan it is Retenc*ion* or suffocac*ion*. or p*re*cipitac*ion* of fflouris they ben alwey. black or livid*us*. but þo þ*at* com of p*re*cipitac*ion*. or suffocac*ion* ben lesse þan they þ*at* Com of Retencioun of fflourys. and tho //that\\ peryn i*n* vrym of hiȝ colo*ur*. *and* Riȝt smal þo Com of p*re*cipitac*ion*. of the mat*ri*ce. Egidi*us*. Gordian*us*. & Io*h*anes d*e* *sancto* a*mando*.

poring owt of sede of man or woman onwilful aȝens kind Ysaac.

¶ And if it apper wan and w*ith* remyshnes and thyn it tokneth gomore of feblenes Ysaac.

¶ Also asshis in vrin tokneth disese of the splen / of the mat*ri*ce, of themraud*is*, and shal not discerne oon from another be colour ffor whan it is retention or suffocation or precipitation of flour*is* thei be alwai blac or liuid*us*, but the{y} that cu*m* of precipitation or suffocation be les than thei that cum of retention of flouris, and the{y} that pere in vrin of hie colour, and right smal thei cu*m* of p*re*cipitation of the matrice Egidius Gordia*nus* Et Io*hanes*. de s*ancto*. a*mando*.

Ipostasys. sedymen. Nefilis. Norma.
Informat sedimen color. & s*u*bstancia te*mpus*.
Forma locus. color e*st* alb*us* s*u*bsta*n*cia gunifis.
Co*n*tinua suis. conu*m* sua forma figurat.
Inferior locus fu*n*dus substancia tempus.
//¶\\ Albu*m* continu*um* Residens *con*stans pineatu*m*.
Si sedimen fiat. bona fit digestio v*irtus*.

¶ to this Ipostasis shulde long. v. *con*diciou*n*s that is to sey. his colo*ur*. his s*u*bstau*n*ce. his place. his tyme. his shappe. The. i. it must be white of Colo*ur* forwhi. ffor the me*m*bris radical. i*n* her*e* disposicio*u*n firste

f. 42r wer*e* whitte. if ypostasis be | nat white. it betokenyth onhelthe. The. 2. is þ*at* his substau*n*ce shulde be holl and nat flettyn*g* then is þe. thryd digestion good. *and* per*f*ecte w*ith*outte ve*n*tosite. for whan it brekyth. and goyth in clowtys heir*e* and þ*er*. then it betoken*yth* ventosite in. 3. digestion. The. 3. co*n*diciou*n* is his. place that he shulde. abyde in þe

To the ypostasis shuld long v condicions that is to say, his colour, his substans, his place, his tyme, his shap. ¶ The first. it shuld be white of colour, ffor whi, ffor the membres radical in her disposition first were white, Yf yposta*sis* be not white it tokneth onhelth ¶ The second is that his substans shul be hole and not fleting. then is the third digestion good and p*er*fecte w*ith*oute ventosite for when it brekith and goth in cloutis here and ther then it tokneth ventosite in the thirde digestion The third, is his place, that he shuld abide in the botom

beneth | ¶ The 4 is his tyme that is last f. 20r
long and many days it tokneth strenght of kinde ¶ The. 5. is his shap, that it be like a pyn apyl white clere / and the brode ende to the botom of thurynal if it be co*n*trary it tokneth onhelth Galen.

3218 remyshnes] *cancel.* remyshynes | **3228** þat] *cancel.* they | **3238** locus] *cancel.* e*st* | **3240** sedimen] *cancel.* sedime

3221 matrice] *ext. marg.* mat*rice* | **3237** Continua] *corr. by exp. and suprascr.* continua/ta\ *m.r.* | **3238** locus fundus] *transp.* fu*n*dus loc*us* *m.r.* | substancia] *corr. by exp. and suprascr.* /con\stancia *m.r.* | **3240** virtus] *ext. marg. etcetera* | **3244** i] *ext. marg.* .i. | **3248** 2] *int. marg.* .2. | **3255** 3^2] *int. marg.* .3.

2706 cloutis] *cancel.* clouthis

2680 asshis] *ext. marg.* ¶ Asshis./

¶ Eu*ery* black Ipostasis is nat for to dreden for somtyme it apperyth black
f. 43v because of | Malencoly. and þ*a*t is Co*m*myn*ly* in dissoluy*ng* þ*er*of as in Co*m*myng of a feu*er* qu*ar*teyn. and also in d*ri*yng or stoppyng of þe ffIourys. or of brestyng outt of þe flouris aft*er* þe drying of hem. and som/tyme\ Ipostasis is black because of adustio*un* and somtyme because of Mortificac*ion*. in þe. ij. firste it betokenyth warysshyng. the. ij. laste wysis. betoken deth. for if Ipostasis be black because of adustion. kyndly hete is consuptt to þe ffulle. and it be black because of Mortificac*ion*. kyndly hete is que*n*chyd and consuptt throuh malice of mat*er* of þe maledy *con*stantin*um*. 7°.

¶ also Ipostasis like b*ro*me betokenyth of þe bladd*er*. and whan it is black or grene if it be in þe botom it is wers þan it wer*e* in þe myddys. and whan it stantt nat Iust i*n* þe botom but fletyth. it betokenyth þ*a*t digestion is hurt þrouh moch wynde auycen*na*. & Gordian*us*.

¶ also yf þe Ipostasis be broke and houe in þe myddys or. aboue it betokenyth bad dygestion and coldnes of þe lyu*er*. and it aper*e* brenny it is evyl. and yf it apper*e* scaly it wersse anamely if þey be whit. *and* sofft. *and* smoth Gor*dianus*

f. 44r ¶ also loke weth*er* þe substau*n*ce be thycke or thynne. or betwyn bothe. ¶ and þe vryn be thy*n*ne þu shalt se through the vryn þe Ioyntis of thi ffyngris. and þ*a*t thy*n*nhed betokenyth. a bad spleen. and a bad stomak. *and* wat*er* in þe bowell*is*. ysaac.

¶ and if þe vryn be thycke that þu mayst nat se through. than it betokenyth wynde in þe stomak. *and* in þe hed and. i*n* þe bowell*is*. ysaac.

¶ and if it {be} betwyn thycke and thy*n*ne then it betokenyth swellyng of þe galle. ysaac.

. 20. *contenta*. Syntilla. or Sparklis.

¶ Syntylla they ben lyke smale

3361 brestyng] *cancel.* up | **3390** betwyn] *cancel.* bethwyn

3375 and] *ext. marg.* Rew*le* | **3390** thynne] *ext. marg.* thy*n*ne | **3397** thycke] *ext. marg.* thicke

it be in the botom it is wors than whan it is in the mydd*is* and whan it standith not iust in the botom but fletith it tokneth that digestion is hurt thorow moch wind Auic*enna* Gord*ianus*.

¶ Yf the iposta*sis* be broke or houe in the mydd*is* or above it tokneth bad digestion and coldnes of the lyuer And it aper bre*n*ny it is evil and it aper scali it is worse and namely if thei be white and softe and smoth Gord*ianus*.//

¶ Also loke whether the substans be thik or thyn or betwen both ¶ And thurin be thyn thow shalt se thorow thi ioynt*is* of the fyngers and that thynhede betokneth a bad splen and a bad stomoc and water in the bowell*is* Ysaac.

¶ And if thuryn be thik that thow maist not se thorow than it tokneth wind in the stomoc and in thede, and in the bowell*is* Ysaac.

¶ And if it be betwen thik and thyn it tokneth swelling of the gal Ysaac

SINTILLA. thei be like smal sp*ar*kill*is* of fyre and thei go downward and vpward in the medil region the wich is cleped the region p*er*forate, and it tokneth the stomoc is ful of wicked

sp*ar*klys. of fyr*e*. and they goon downward. upward in þe mydel region. þe wech is clepyd þe regi{on} p*er*forat. and it betokenyth þe stomak is full of wyckyd hum*er*is. and disposyd to spue. Gordian*us*.

¶ vryn in an hote accesse. black. *and* litell qua*n*tyte. ffatte and stynkyng. morte*m* sig*nifica*t.

¶ vryn in an hote accesse on p*ar*ty Red anoþ*er* p*ar*ty black. or grene. or blew. morte*m* sig*nifica*t.

¶ vryn ou*er* all keu*er*yd w*ith* led. or like touh betokenyth. a prolongacio*u*n of deth.

¶ vryn derke. above. and cler*e* benethe f. 44v | betokenyth deth.

¶ vryn that shewyth hi*m*selff riȝtt cler*e*. *and* bryȝt. and þe skye. i*n* þe botom shynat. morte*m* sig*nifica*t.

//¶\\ vryn thyn of s*u*bstau*n*ce hauy*n*g or fletyng aboue. as. a derke skye. morte*m* sig*nifica*t.

¶ vryn d*ra*sty stynkyng. *and* black skye w*i*th*y*nne betokenyth. a p*ro*longacio*u*n toward deth.

//¶\\ vryn þ*a*t is like wat*er*. yf it haue a derke skye in an accesse. morte*m*. sig*nifica*t./

¶ vryn þ*a*t hayþ d*ra*stys in þe botom medlyd w*ith* blood betokenyt deth./

¶ vryn black. and thy*n*ne if þe pacient be loth to speke. or yf he vnd*er*stond nat. or if his Issu wil nat goo from hi*m*. morte*m* sig*nifica*t./

¶ vryn. black i*n* a feu*er* w*ith*. a spume if his nose blede. morte*m* sig*nificat*./

//¶\\ vryn. i*n*. a feu*er* yf it t*ur*ne like mylke. morte*m* sig*nificat*./

¶ vryn trobly þ*a*t hayþ holdyng cloddys. abovyn fletyn. morte*m* sig*nifica*t./

//¶\\ vryn like blood. w*ith* akyng at þe h*er*te. þe hed veyne betyng on þe riȝtt side. morte*m* sig*nifica*t./

¶ vryn white w*ith*out substau*n*ce. and above*n* haþ moch spume. morte*m* sig*nifica*t./

//¶\\ vryn þ*a*t haþ flesh and heyr*e*. þe

humours and disposed to spew Gord*ianus*./

¶ Vryn in an hote axes blac and litil in qua*n*tite and stinking morte*m* sig*nifica*t

¶ Vrin in an hote axes on p*ar*ty red anoth*er* p*ar*ty blac or gren or blew morte*m* s*ignifica*t

¶ Vrin al keuerd ou*er* w*ith* lede or like touȝh tokneth a prolongation of deth

¶ Vryn derke above | and clere beneth f. 21r tokneth deth

¶ Vryn that shewith hy*m*self right clere and bright and the skye in the botom shyneth morte*m* sig*nifica*t

¶ Vryn thyn of substans hoving or fleting above as a dark skye mortem sig*nifica*t

¶ Vryn drasty stinking, and blac skye w*ith*in tokneth a prolongation toward deth

¶ Vryn like water, if it haue a darke skye in an axes, mortem sig*nifica*t

¶ Vrin w*ith* drast*is* in the botom medled w*ith* blode tokneth deth

¶ Vrin blac and thyn if the pacient be loth to speke, or if he vnd*er*stond not, or if his Ischew wil not go from hym morte*m* sig*nifica*t

¶ Vrin blac in a feuer w*ith* a spume, if his nose blede morte*m* sig*nifica*t

¶ Vrin trobly that hath holding clodd*is* above fleting. morte*m* sig*nifica*t

¶ Vrin in a feuer if it turn lik mylke morte*m* sig*nifica*t

¶ Vryn like blode w*ith* aking at tharte, thede, veyn betyng on the right side morte*m* sig*nifica*t

¶ Vrin white and w*ith*out substanc*e* and above hath moch spume morte*m* sig*nificat*.

¶ Vrin that hath flesh or here the bladd*er* is scabby and tokneth long siknes or deth

¶ Vryn blac and Watry in a fat man. Mortes significat.///

3445 holdyng] *cancel.* g

bladd*er* is scaby. *and* betokenyth long siknes. or deth./

¶ vryn black. *and* wat*ri*. i*n*. a fatt man. morte*m* sig*nifica*t.

3458 significat] *bot. marg.* The end of the Treatise of Urines *m.r.*

2.3. English translation of Giles de Corbeil's *Carmen de urinis* in MS Hunter 328

15 de … 34 formis]
Concerning black urine: the first chapter
A rather dark aspect of urine [indicates] a troublesome fever
[if] it weakens in a four-day cycle; [if] it burns, it signals death;
if it settles black to the base [of the vessel], the humour checks itself.
[If] the womb is purged, [there is] a draining of much flux;
in a black fever it brings death, [but] little stink
after the damage to the bladder and the kidneys are completely removed.
On many a day, critically, a black hanging cloudiness
grows largely dark and disturbs the floating sediment,
and it is disturbed when the ears are vexed [and] there is a lack of sleep.
It indicates that a bloody flux will come from the nose,
but if it combines the bad signs without [hope] of salvation,
it condemns with a verdict of death, or [otherwise] frees the sick one
in keeping suitable agreements with the density of the mixture.
A slight darkness of liquid recoils from coitus
when it tolerates a thinness which does not remain matching in colour,
[but] produces an outcome and causes violent results
[when the urine] is not slightly blocked, [and the] drawing-off from the channels is closed.
Twice ten colours can be distinguished in urine,
which you can assess through the forms written here.

276 contra … 296 color]
Against the power of death, there is no medicine in the gardens.
Concerning livid urine, the colour of which is the colour of lead.
Urine is grey-blue if there is lividity or partial lividity:
collect the various causes for the leaden colour of urine;
either there will be total bruising throughout every limb
or it indicates that the humour of the limb is mortified,
or in addition [such a] livid urine fits various causes:
mild, semitertian, middling sickness, middling fleeting,
continuous abdominal dropsy, a burst vein, catarrh,
stranguries, the collapse of the womb, the suffering of flux,
some defect in the rib or lung, arthritic pain,
consumptive tuberculosis scarcely reducing in heat,
let these be causes for lividity as far as you are concerned: collect them through signs.
A thin trickle [of urine], barely combined, livid, oily [signifies] death;

[Such a] continuous [urine] presages a boy or a young man
dominated by gall when healthy, and signs him with its own mark.
A quartan erratic fever has marked out such a one
rather in autumn and in the hours of winter;
it speaks to damage the chest, the spleen, the liver,
an offense to the breast, [and, when] linked to connected particles,
the spleen. If it shines variegated with many stripes,
a large effusion of liquid shows a dry liver;
in a continual fever, such as under the light of disease,
when it is prolonged, it badly brings in a loss of vigour
at the middle-point, [but] frenzy just before the end of the fight.
It designates that critically the signs of calming of phlegm are strengthening,
and with the bile which it compounds with wine, it renders
[the urine] lemon-yellow, thin, the humour bordering on lemon.
When rough, [the urine is] thinner, and when smooth, less thin.
[It is] more intense with a fever, [but] diminished without a fever.

1398 In ... 1438 fidelis]
Turning to red-gold, the colour is clearly close to that of gold.
[When] level, middling, pure to the [colour], the liquid matches
in a phlegmatic boy, a youth, an old man, a woman.
[Urine that] stays red-gold [and] thin indicates the disagreeableness of a fever;
when continuous, or tertian or duplex, but in a long period,
damage to the liver, or a four-day fever
at the beginning of the symptoms, while there are the new seeds of sickness.
Red-gold, slightly thin, the topmost part of the section of which
a loose cloud occupies, produced by the motion of heat,
[such urine] enflames a swelling fever from salty phlegm
but it figures a tertian fever when the sickness is already in progress.
[Urine is just] a little dense, now [signals] not a tertian fever, [but] rather a one-day [fever],
a fever with unsalty or sweet phlegm.
[If] the biting humour [that comes] from salty phlegm is abundant
and had come without fever: that excites mighty movements,
being extreme, striking the parts with the sharpness of fervour.
If [the urine is] slightly red-gold, a little thin, [and] it does not turn out cloudy,
but it keeps such a form for a constant time,
such [a liquid] is reckoned fatal for one suffering from dropsy.
[If the urine is] a bit red-gold, oily, retaining cloudy shading,
it shows that a fever is enflamed from sweet phlegm,
the heat subsists within, or the substance is there,
an outflowing of sweet phlegm is indicated without fever.

[If the urine is] a bit red-gold, oily, livid, constant,
[it indicates that] the organs in which breathing occurs with sweet phlegm
or with saltiness, it shows with a certain reasoning that they grow heavy;
in a woman it rather indicates a disturbance in the womb.
If the colour is red-gold and [there is] an oily substance in the vessel where [the urine] is kept, it indicates a continual fever [arising] from phlegm.
If that is a recent symptom, and the lividity darkens the topmost area,
either a lesser [fever] is indicated, or pleurisy is implied;
if it is an old [symptom], abdominal dropsy rather, or it is called an abscess,
if it turns out more frothy, and of the colour of ash,
rheumatic, a weak organ with a distressing complaint,
it could be considered oily, or it could be of a red-gold colour;
if it turns out more frothy, and of the colour of ash
somewhat distinctly livid, red-gold, slack,
the sickness migrates to the areas of the lung and side;
[if it is] greasy, red-gold, a bit livid, oily, [with signs of] filament,
[it is] linked to hectic fever, [and is] a sure sign.

1604 Clara … 1617 monstrat]
Clear, ruddy [urine indicates] a six-day fever, or an overheated liver
and can imply a quartan swelling.
This is a delay, or brevity, cloud, time, status, age;
the suffering, form, place of the sick one proves this.
In order that the diagnosis proceeds on a stable footing there are these things:
all are to be discussed in your judgement.
[Whether the urine is] murky, dense, slightly steeped in a ruddy colour,
continuous, tertian, [it is] surely presented as harmful.
If a greenness reaches the top, or [there is] a livid cloud,
it presages a middling or pleuritic ailment.
Dense, ruddy [urine means] a continuous fever if the lividity shadows the top;
dense, ruddy, it signals a continuous fever when the lividity has disappeared;
It means burning fever if it is thinner than it has turned dense;
fine and fiery [urine] indicates continuous burning fever.

1876 Si … 1882 immoderatus]
If the colour is wine-faced, it means harm to health,
[and that will be] continuous with fever; it is less to be feared without fever,
for the hot humour burns the kidneys or the liver;
it is either chyle that has erupted, or is seeping from a broken vessel,
[or] menstrual blood is drawn from a woman's body.
Vigorous movement produces such a thing in a healthy body
or too much sex or purging or immoderate effort.

1912 Non … 1914 virore]
The blue colour [of urine] is not debased, according to the law of an earlier man;
[it means] jaundice, major cramp and, finally, death;
urine tinged with leek-green verdancy offers a diagnosis.

2211 Sepius … 2238 utrumque]
Quite often the form of the colour fools the craftsman:
the assessment of the liquid beguiles the faith of many.
In the contents there is confirmed law [and] sure distinction:
the constant rule of judgement, true faith.
Setting aside the rest, the canny author on nature,
Hippocras, draws from here the true seeds of truth.
Now let the form of the contents be noted in order,
And let what is noted keep its own properties:
(1) ring (2) bubble (3) grain (4) cloud (5) froth
(6) pus (7) oiliness (8) chyme (9) blood (10) grit (11) hair
(12) scales (13) flakes (14) mealiness (15) tiny specks
(16) sperm (17) ash (18) sediment (19) substance (20) spark.
If the ring in the urine is thick and watery,
the rear cell, when pressed, aches with phlegm.
[If it is] thick, purple, it mainly afflicts the blood
[but if it is] pale, thin, [it afflicts] the left [side] with black bile.
The intensity of the fevered one will be with choler on the right-hand side
if the thin ring is lemon-yellow or ruddy in colour.
Lead-coloured [liquid] suggests that the root of feeling
is dying, and that the damages also spread to the branches
if, after first seeming livid, it later seems ruddy.
The nature of the power of the brain surges and is recovered
if it takes on the form and the strength of causon in the fever.
A humour of gall is inflamed to the stirring of frenzy
if it is quivering; the organs of the back are afflicted
if it appears dark or mortifying or is burning:
the preceding strength or lividity distinguishes each of the two.

2308 Non … 2318 debiliorem]
A swelling bubble that does not remain, sticking together gassily,
makes fresh the cause of sickness, and the sickness that it causes to grow,
and it produces kidney disease and damages the brain with aching,
and causes roaring vomit and an aching of the stomach.

2352 Granula … 2357 debiliorem]
'Grains'; particles
Small particles are always the indicator of a condition of watery discharge.
If the small granules are deposited in a circular arrangement,

then the hidden confusion of sickness is concealed in the brain;
If they are underlying and barely detected, and do not change back,
they will hasten; the humour attacks the places closest to the head,
[and] the flux ends up lower down, towards the weaker area.

2375 …2377 calorem]
Little cloud; 'a cloud'; cloud
A little cloudiness in an airy form indicates
firmly a fault of a spiritual organ, and the heat of the liver.

2427 … 2435 croco]
'Froth'. 'Scum'. Froth.
[If] the froth is gassy, or perhaps of intense colour,
it is an indicator when combined with its own particles.
The colour of the urine proves this, [and] its essence, and froth:
the vapour thickens and the heat diminishes.
Variegated [urine], distinct with tiny particles
strikes the organs weak with the particle with rheum;
it points to jaundice or presages that the liver becomes enflamed
if it is dark or green or tinged with saffron colouring.

2520 … 2524 probat]
Pus 'Pus'. 'Quitter', Poison. 'It is all the same'.
Pus pouring out [in urine] speaks to the sores of a blister
or an eruption of the kidneys if a strong smell is present.
The suppurating sediment comes to an end from the area of the liver;
the pain and damaged action of that organ prove that.

2614 … 2616 febre[2]]
Spider's web. Fat. Greasy [urine]. 'Fatness'.
[Urine] presenting with an oily appearance [or] a fatty solution
with a fever dissolves the whole [body], [just the] loins in the absence of fever.

2689 … 2693 suppremus]
Humour. Chyme. 'Raw humour'. Raw humour.
As for the humour in urine: if the topmost part is undigested food in suspension,
it causes harm to the highest limbs, but the middle or lowest part
produces strangury, [and] if it persists, frenzy and hallucination;
the middle part afflicts the digestive [organs], the top the midriff.

2766 blood … 2777 daturus]
'Blood'. Blood.
The presence of gore [in urine] stems from damage of the liver,
of the bladder, of the kidneys, of the vein, of chyle; this is plenty for you.

3. Glossary

3.1. Conventions

This section contains a selected glossary of the Middle English terms in *H*, the source used as the base text for the present edition. As this volume is ultimately designed for an academic readership, the present glossary includes lexical words such as nouns (*n.*),[1] adjectives (*a.*), verbs (*v.*) and adverbs (*adv.*),[2] disregarding those words which a Middle English scholar is surely familiar with, mostly grammatical words like determiners, pronouns, prepositions and conjunctions. The underlying impulse here is, therefore, the compilation of lexical words, both general and scientific, to offer an *ad hoc* tool for a successful reading of the text. Proper names have also been recorded so as to help the reader in the understanding of the medical practitioner involved in each case.

The entry structure sequentially displays the following information: a) the headword; b) the part of speech; c) the meaning of the glossed items. In addition, the different variant forms are also alphabetically listed together with the number of occurrences in H328.

Several conventions have been used in the layout of the entries. Headwords are given in bold type reproducing the most frequent spelling in the text. The different suffixal forms of a same base are given as headwords as in the case of the adjectives *oyly* and *oylysh*, which share the same semantic connotations denoting the meaning of 'oilish, resembling oil'. For convenience, both forms are given independent entries in the glossary so as to provide additional information about the diffusion of these suffixes in combination with that particular base.

Exceptionally, however, we make room for particular grammatical items when their spelling is not fully transparent, thus not easily identifiable with its corresponding lemma. If a word shows an obscure allograph, hence not

[1] Verbal nouns, in turn, are noted with the abbreviation (*ng.*).

[2] Adverbs, in turn, are often fuzzily interpreted as to whether they are, strictly speaking, lexical or grammatical words. The glossary is restricted to listing adjuncts of manner insofar as, unlike other adverb types, they semantically modify the action expressed by the verb.

easily identifiable with its corresponding headword, we grant it the status of a headword to refer back to its factual lemma. For instance, the noun *postym* 'a morbid swelling or inflammation in any part of the body' is variously rendered by the scribe both with and without the prefixal form *em-* (i.e. *postym* and *empostym*), these being problematic to associate for a reader not familiar with Middle English medical lore. For this reason, the prefixed form *empostym* has been also recorded referring the reader to the headword *postym*, where all the semantic and grammatical information of this term is contained. For simplicity, the symbol (>) has been used for these purposes. In this vein, the entry empostym > postym, *n.* refers to the factual headword postym.

Part-of-speech tags, on the other hand, are italicised in the glossary by using the following notation: nouns (*n.*), adjectives (*adj.*), verbs (*v.*) and adverbs (*adv.*). The word class becomes an added asset here to disambiguate lexical items with the same headword, as in the case of *syke, adj.* and *syke, n.* or *grose, adj.* and *grose, n.*

Meanings, in turn, are partially reproduced according to the definition found in the *e-MED* (Kurath et al. 2001) and the *Oxford English Dictionary* (Simpson, Edmund and Weiner 1989). These sources, however, are not always reliable in regard to uroscopy terms and, for that reason, in many cases an in-text definition is provided taken from these sources and other uroscopy treatises. These readings have been also supported by other specific dictionaries such as Norri's recent *Dictionary of Medical Vocabulary in English, 1375–1550: Body Parts, Sicknesees, Instruments, and Medicinal Preparations* (2016) as well as the *Dictionary of Medieval Latin from British Sources* (Latham, Howlett and Ashdowne (1975–), the latter for Latinate and Greek terms in particular. If a particular tag phrase, collocation or prepositional verb deserves mentioning, these appear at the end of the corresponding entry preceded by two horizontal bars where the implicit lemma has been shortened for the sake of brevity. For instance, the adjective *nutrityf* 'nutritious' displays the noun phrase *membres nutritives* with the following arrangement: || membres ~, 'organs whose function is to nourish the body, nutritive members'.

Given the level of spelling variation in Middle English, the entries also contain the complete set of variant forms together with their occurrences. These variants are arranged in terms of frequency, distinguishing the different abbreviated (and underlined) forms of each spelling for further linguistic research.

A

abrode, *adv.* Scattered over a large area, widely
abrode (1×)

absteynen, *v.* To avoid (sth.); refrain from partaking of (food, etc.)
absteyn*e* (1×)

abyden, *v.* To remain, stay; to experience or undergo (pain, hardship), suffer
abyde (2×), abydyng (1×), abydyth (1×)

accesse, *n.* An attack of illness characterised by fever, especially of ague
accesse (8×), acesse (1×), excesse (1×)

acetosum, *adj.* Sour, acid
Acetosu*m* (1×), acetosu*m* (3×)

acorden, *v.* To be compatible or harmonious
acordyth (1×)

acthe, *n.* Ache
acthe (6×), ach (4×), ache (1×), ach*e* (1×), Ackth (1×), akthe (1×)

admixtion, *n.* The act or process of mingling, mixing together; the condition of being mingled or mixed
admixtio*ne*ȝ (1×)

aduste, *adj.* Morbidly altered in nature by the action of the heat of the body
aduste (4×)

adustion, *n.* Cauterisation; the corruption of bodily humours, ulcers, etc. by heat
adustion (7×), adustio*u*n (6×), adustiu*n* (1×), adustyon (6×), adustyo*u*n (1×), adusty*u*n (1×), adustyun (1×)

aforeseyd, *adj.* Aforesaid
afor*e*seyd (4×), aforseyd (2×)

afforismus, *n.* Aphorism
aff*orismus* (2×), afforysm*us* (1×)

age, *n.* Age
agys (1×)

agu, *n.* Acute fever, or an attack of it
agu (9×)

akthe > **acthe**, *n.*

akyng, *ng.* Pain, aching
akyng (3×), hakyng (1×)

alba, *adj.* Clear, white as water of a well
alba (3×), alba (1×), Albe (1×), albi (1×), alb*us* (1×)

alchites, *n.* A collection of serous fluid in the peritoneal cavity; dropsy of the abdomen; ascites
alchites (2×)

ale, *n.* Beer, ale
ale (5×)

aloe epatyk, *n.* An opaque, liver-coloured form of Socotrine aloes; exhibiting minute crystals of Aloin
aloe Epatyk (1×), aloen epatyk (1×), aloes epatyk (1×)

altherworst, *adj.* Worst of all
alth*er*worst (1×)

alyenacioun, *n.* Derangement, insanity
alyenacio*u*n (2×), alyenac*i*on (2×), alyenanc*i*on (1×)

ampulla, *n.* Dilation, swelling, one of the standard uroscopic contents, defined as *burbyl* ‘bubble’ or a *bolme* (not in MED, probably a nominal form of *bolnen* v. or *bolni* adj.)
ampulla (2×), ampull*e* (1×)

ampullous, *adj.* Bubbly, having bubbles
a*m*pullosa (1×)

amydown, *n.* Crushed hulled wheat; grits, starch
amydown (1×)

bloo, *adj.* Leaden, livid, greyish colour
Bloo (19×)

blood, *n.* Blood
blood (39×), blod (5×), blod (1×)

bloody, *adj.* With blood
bloody (1×)

bloones, *n.* Lividness
bloones (2×)

blooysh, *adj.* Leaden, greyish
blooysh (2×)

bocche, *n.* Any pathological swelling
bocchys (1×)

bodily, *adj.* Bodily
bodily (1×)

body, *n.* The human body
body (71×), bodyes (2×), body (1×)

boke, *n.* Book
boke (3×)

bolme, *n.* A bubble
bolme (1×), bolmys (1×)

bolnen, *v.* To swell (from infection)
bolne (2×), bolny*n* (1×), bolnyth (1×)

bolnyng, *ng.* Swelling, distention
bolny*n*g (2×)

borage, *n.* Borage
borag*e* (1×), borage (1×)

bore, *n.* An uncastrated male swine
bore (1×)

botom, *n.* The lower part or side of something; base, foundation, bottom
botom (18×), botym (13×), botu*m* (5×), bottom (2×), bottu*m* (2×)

bowel, *n.* A human intestine
bowell*is* (4×)

boylen, *v.* To cook by boiling; prepare (remedies or their ingredients) by boiling
boyle (2×), boylyd (1×)

brain, *n.* The brain
brayn (8×), brayn (1×), baryn (1× *poss. error*)

bran > **bren**, *n.*

brayen, *v.* To mix ingredients by stamping in a mortar
bray (1×)

bred, *n.* Bread
bred (4×), brede (1×)

breden, *v.* To breed, generate, give rise to
bred (2×)

bredyng, *ng.* Hatching, incubation; gestation
bredyng (1×), bredy*n*g (1×)

breken, *v.* To break into parts; dash to pieces
breke (3×), brekyth (1×), broke (3×), broken (2×), brokyn (3×)

brekyng, *ng.* The act or fact of the breaking, crushing, or tearing
brekyng (5×)

bren, *n.* Bran
bren (5×), bran (2×), brenn (1×)

brennen, *v.* To be consumed by fire; burn; to alter or corrupt with body heat
brent (3×), brentt (1×)

brenny, *adj.* Bran-like
bre*n*ny (2×), brenny (1×)

brennyng, *ng.* A burning sensation; inflammation, festering; cauterisation
bre*n*ny*n*g (8×), brenny*n*g (2×)

brest, *n.* Breast; chest
brest (10×), breste (10×), breste (1×)

bresten, *v.* To be broken, fall apart, break
broste (1×)

brestyng, *ng.* The bursting of a boil, ulcer, etc.; an eruption of pimples; hernia
brestyng (3×)

breth, *n.* Breathing
breth (9×), breth (1×)

brethyd, *adj.* Having respiration
brethyd (1×)

breue, *n.* Porridge, pulse; broth (of meat), liquor (of vegetables)
breues (1×)

brode, *adj.* Wide, broad
brode (2×)

brom, *n.* Broom
brom (1×), b*rome* (1×)

brotylnesse, *n.* Fragility; weakness, feebleness
brotylnesse (1×)

bryȝt, *adj.* Clear, bright
bryȝt (6×), bryȝtt (6×), briȝtt (2×)

bryȝtnesse, *n.* Brightness, brilliance, radiance
bryȝtnesse (1×), bryhtnesse (1×)

bugle, *n.* A blue-flowered herb of the mint family
bugle (1×)

burble, *n.* A bubble
burblys (7×), burbyl (1×)

buttok, *n.* A buttock
butokk*is* (2×)

byden, *v.* To stay, remain
byde (2×), bydeth (1×)

byndyng, *adj.* Sticky, glutinous, adherent
by*n*dyng (1×)

C

cacchen, *v.* To catch, grasp, seize
cauȝt (1×)

calamyntte, *n.* The common calamint
Calamy*n*tte (1×)

calculus, *n.* A small stone, pebble
Calcul*us* (1×)

caleffaccioun, *n.* An inflammation
caleffacci*oun* (1×)

calle, *n.* An enveloping membrane
Calle (1×)

callen, *v.* To call, name
calle (1×), callyd (15×)

canel, *n.* Cinnamon
canel (1×)

care, *n.* The pain of disease or death
care (1×)

cassia fistula, *n.* Pods of the tree cassia fistula; also, the pulp from these pods
cassia ffistula (1×), cassia fistula (1×)

casten, *v.* To utter; heave
caste (1×)

castyng, *ng.* Urination, especially for the purposes of examination
castyng (1×)

cathalempcia, *n.* Catalepsy, a seizure, with loss of sensation and consciousness
Cathalempcia (1×)

cause, *n.* Cause
cause (5×), causis (1×), causys (1×)

causen, *v.* To cause, effect or produce (sth.)
cause (1×), causyd (21×), causyth (3×)

causon, *n.* A kind of chronic fever, burning fever
causon (1×)

celidonie, *n.* The greater celandine; any of its parts used medicinally
Celidonie (1×)

centory, *n.* The common centaury
Centory (1×)

cerkyl, *n.* A geometrical circle
cerkyl (27×), c*er*kyl (8×)

certeyn, *adj.* Certain
*cer*teyn (1×), certeyn (1×)

chafyng, *ng.* Morbid heat, inflammation
chafyng (1×)

change, *n*. Alteration, variation, change
change (1×)
changeabyl, *adj*. Subject to variation or change; variable, unstable
changeabyl (1×)
changen, *v*. To change
chong (1×), choyngyn (1×)
chapter, *n*. Chapter, a division in a piece of writing
chapt*er* (1×), Chaptrys (1×)
chiken, *n*. A young chicken; chick, pullet
Chikenes (1×)
child, *n*. Child, baby
chyld (4×), chylde (3×), chyldryn (1×)
chimus, *n*. Chyme, undigested food, the semifluid pulpy acid matter into which food is converted in the stomach by the action of the gastric secretion. From the stomach it passes into the small intestine, and by the action on it of the bile becomes fitted for absorption as chyle
chimus (2×)
chyncok, *n*. Syncope, loss of consciousness accompanied by weakening of the pulse
Chy*n*cok (1×)
chyneboon, *n*. The bone of the lower jaw, jawbone
Chyneboon (1×)
chyppyng, *ng*. Clippings, fragments
chyppyng (1×)
chysel, *n*. Gravel, sand
chysel (2×), schysell*is* (1×)
ciner, *n*. Ashes
Cineris (1×), Cin*er*is (1×)
cirage, *n*. A form of gout in the joints of the hand
Cirage (1×)
citrine, *adj*. Reddish or brownish yellow, as a yellow apple
Cit*r*ine (19×), Cit*r*ine (2×), citrina (1×), cit*r*ine (1×), cit*r*inor*um* (1×), citryn (1×), citryne (1×)
clensyng, *ng*. Capacity for cleansing or for purging
clensyng (1×)
clepen, *v*. To name
clepyd (10×), clepyd (1×)
clere, *adj*. Not turbid; transparent, translucent
cler*e* (15×), clere (5×)
clernes, *n*. Brightness; shininess
clernes (1×)
cleuen, *v*. To stick, adhere
cleue (1×), Cleuyth (1×)
cley, *n*. Any argillaceous earth; clay
cley (1×)
clod, *n*. A lump of earth or clay, a clod
cloddys (1×)
clodden, *v*. To coagulate, clot
cloddyd (1×), Cloddyn (1×)
cloddy, *adj*. Full of clots, thrombotic
cloddy (1×)
close, *adv*. Tightly, firmly, securely
close (1×)
clote, *n*. The common burdock
clot*is* (1×)
cloth, *n*. A piece of woven or felted fabric; a cloth
cloth (2×)
cloudy, *adj*. Opaque; smoky; dim
cloudy (2×)
cloutty, *adj*. Full of curds
cloutty (1×)
clowde, *n*. An accumulation of clouds, mist, or fog; a cloud
clowde (9×), cloutt*is* (4×), cloude (2×), clowdy (1×), clowdys (1×)
clowt, *n*. A fragment or piece
clowtt*is* (1×), clowtys (1×)
cobweb, *n*. Spiderweb, cobweb
Cobweb (1×)
codde, *n*. Crop, craw; belly
codde (2×)

cold, *adj.* Cold
cold (18×), Cold (1×), colde (1×)
coldnesse, *n.* Coldness
coldnesse (4×), coldnes (1×)
coler > **colour**, *n.*
coler, *n.* Bile, one of the four primary humours
col*er* (16×), col*er*a (6×), Col*er* (4×), coler (3×), col*er*is (1×), col*er*ram (1×), Colr*e* (1×), colr*e* (1×)
colerryk, *adj.* Of body fluids: characterised by excessive or toxic colre
col*er*ryk (3×), Col*er*ica (1×), coleryk (1×), coleryk (1×), col*er*yk (1×), colryk (1×)
colica passio, *n.* Disease affecting the colon; suffering with colic
Colica passio (2×), Colica passio (1×), colica passyo (1×), colyca passyo (1×)
colleccion, *n.* The action or process of gathering
collecc*io*n (1×)
colour, *n.* Colour
colo*ur* (62×), colour (6×), colour*e* (5×), colo*ur* (2×), coloris (2×), col*er* (1×), col*er* (1×), colo*ur* (1×), colour*es* (1×), colours (1×), colourys (1×)
colouren, *v.* To make (sth.) a certain colour
colo*ur*d (1×)
colre > **coler**, *n.*
columbyn, *n.* The columbine
Colu*m*byn (1×)
colyk, *n.* A disease characterised by severe abdominal pain, the colic
Colyk (2×), Colik (1×)
comen, *v.* To come
com (45×), comyth (39×), comyn (5×), cu*m* (2×), co*m*myth (1×), comyng (1×), com*y*t*h* (1×)
commentoure, *n.* Author; commentator
Co*m*me*n*tour*e* (1×)
commyng, *ng.* Arrival, approach, coming
co*m*my*n*g (1×), Co*m*myng (1×)
comyn, *n.* The plant cumin
comyn (1×), co*m*myn (1×)
comynly, *adv.* Jointly, in common; together
comy*n*ly (6×), Co*m*my*n*ly (1×)
compaccion, *n.* Clumpling (together)
compacc*io*n (1×)
company, *n.* Companionship (with the opposite sex)
company (2×)
complexioun, *n.* Constitution or nature resulting from the blending of the four humours
*com*plexio*u*n (2×), *com*plexio*u*ns (1×)
compounyd, *adj.* Mixed, blended; compounded
*com*pounyd (2×), *com*pound (1×), *com*pou*n*yd (1×)
compressyoun, *n.* Exertion of pressure; compressing, squeezing
comp*ressy*o*u*n (1×)
concepcioun, *n.* Conception (of a child)
Concepcio*u*n (1×), co*n*cepci*on* (1×)
condicioun, *n.* A situation or state; condition
co*n*dicio*u*n (1×), *con*dicio*u*ns (1×), *con*dicions (1×)
confeccioun, *n.* Preparation of a medicine by mixing ingredients in a prescribed manner
*con*feccio*u*n (3×)
conffery, *n.* The herb comfrey
co*n*ffery (1×)
congellen, *v.* To solidify in low temperature, freeze
*con*gellyd (1×), congellyd (1×)

dieten, *v.* To regulate the diet for purposes of health
Diet (2×), diete (1×)

digestion, *n.* The digestion of food and drink
digestion (12×), digestio*un* (5×), dygestio*un* (5×), digestyo*un* (3×), dygestion (3×), dygestyon (2×), digestion (1×)

discenterie, *n.* Dysentery
discenterie (1×)

disma, *n.* Laboured or short breathing; dyspnea
disma (1×)

disposen, *v.* To arrange
disposyd (1×), dysposyd (1×), dissposyd (1×)

disposicioun, *n.* Constitution, complexion, or temperament as determined by the blending of humours
disposicio*un* (2×), disposicion (1×), disposycio*un* (1×), dyspocio*un* (1×), dysposysc*io*n (1×), dysposyssio*un* (1×), dyssposicion (1×)

dissernen, *v.* To discriminate, distinguish
dysserne (1×)

disseven, *v.* To deceive (sb.)
dissevyng (1×)

dissoluen, *v.* To break up, dissolve
dissolue (1×)

distemper, *n.* The imbalance of a humour
dystemp*er* (1×)

distemperance, *n.* The imbalance of humours or of qualities
distemp*er*ance (1×)

distemperen, *v.* To suffer the imbalance of a humour
dystemp*er* (1×), dystemp*er*d (1×)

distempure, *n.* A morbid condition; illness; intemperance
distempur*e* (1×), dyste*m*pure (1×)

distynccioun, *n.* The process of discriminating, distinguishing
distynccio*un* (1×)

dobyl, *adj.* Consisting of two like or complementary parts
dobyl (3×), dowbyl (1×)

don, *v.* To do, make; perform
doth (4×), do (2×), dede (1×), doyng (1×)

douctour, *n.* An authority on medicine or surgery, doctor of medicine
douctourys (1×)

drast, *n.* Dregs; sediment, scum
d*ra*stys (1×)

drasty > **dresty**, *a.*

drawen, *v.* To draw (breath), breathe; ~ doun, to drag (sth.) on the ground
drawe (2×), drawyng (2×), draw*yth* (1×), drawyth (1×)

drawyng, *ng.* The action of pulling
drawyng (1×)

drede, *n.* Anxiety, worry, uneasiness
drede (4×)

dreden, *v.* To fear, be afraid of
dreden (1×)

dredful, *adj.* Timid; afraid, frightened
dredfful (1×)

drenchen, *v.* To soak, immerse, drench
drenchyd (1×)

dresty, *adj.* Poor as to colour or quality; like dregs
dresty (2×), d*ra*sty (1×)

droppe, *n.* A drop of liquid
droppys (1×)

dropsye, *n.* The disease, dropsy
dropsye (7×), dropsy (4×), d*ro*psye (4×), d*ro*psy (3×), d*ro*psy (1×), dropsye (1×)

drunkenesse, *n.* The state of being drunk, intoxication
drunkenesse (1×)

drunkyn, *adj.* Drunk, intoxicated
dru*n*kyn (1×)

drye, *adj.* Dry
drye (4×)

dryen, *v.* To dry
drye (1×), dryeth (1×)

drying, *ng.* The act or process of drying; desiccation
drying (3×), dryyng (3×), d*ri*yng (1×), dryeng (1×)

drynes, *n.* The state of being dry or dried out
drynes (7×), drynesse (5×)

drynke, *n.* A beverage, drink
drynke (2×), drynk*is* (2×), drynk (1×), dry*n*k*is* (1×), drynkk*is* (1×)

drynken, *v.* To drink
drynke (5×), d*rinke* (2×), dru*n*kyn (1×), dry*n*k (1×)

drynkyng, *ng.* The action of drinking
drynkyng (3×)

dryven, *v.* To chase, pursue, drive
dryvyth (1×)

dul, *adj.* Incapable of movement or sensation, insensible
dul (1×)

dulnesse, *n.* Bluntness, dullness
dulnesse (1×)

dust, *n.* Dust
dust (1×)

dwellyng, *ng.* The act or fact of residing, residence
dwellyng (1×)

dyabetes, *n.* Diabetes
dyabetes (1×)

dym, *adj.* Dark, dull, dusky
dym (4×), dy*m*me (3×)

dymmen, *v.* To lose brightness, grow dark
dy*m*my*n* (1×)

dymmyng, *ng.* The action of dimming
dy*m*myng (1×)

dymmysh, *adj.* Not bright or shining, dim
dy*m*mysh (1×), dy*m*myssh (1×)

dymnesse, *n.* Dimness, darkness
dy*m*nesse (2×), dy*n*nesse (2×), dy*m*nes (1×)

dysparblen, *v.* To disperse; to dissipate
dysp*ar*blyd (1×)

dyssese, *n.* Suffering, or pain; disease
dyssesys (3×), dissesys (2×), dyssese (2×), dyssesis (1×)

dyssesen, *v.* To hurt or harm bodily; inflict pain
dyssesyd (3×)

dyssire, *n.* Desire
dyssire (1×), dyssyr*e* (1×)

dyssoluyng, *ng.* A solution; disintegration of a solid
dyssoluy*ng* (2×), dissoluy*ng* (1×), dyssoluyng (1×)

dystemperyng, *ng.* The improper balance of the humours or qualities
dystemp*er*yng (1×)

dystrobulance, *n.* Harm, injury
dyst*ro*bulance (1×)

dystroyen, *v.* To destroy
dyst*ro*yd (2×), dist*ro*yed (1×)

dystyllyng, *ng.* Straining, filtering; distillation
dystyllyng (1×)

dyuerse, *adj.* Diverse, various
dyu*er*se (9×), diu*er*se (1×), dyu*ers* (2×)

dyuyden, *v.* To separate into parts; break up, divide
dyuyde (2×), diuydyth (1×)

eg, *n*. Egg
eg (1×)

Egidius, *n*. Giles de Corbeil, a French royal physician (c. 1140–1224)
Egidi*us* (107×), Egidiu*m* (8×), Egidi*us* (6×), Egidi*um* (2×), Edigi*us* (1×), Egid*ium* (1×), Egidiu*m* (1×), Egidi*um* (1×), Egidius (1×)

egre, *adj*. Of pain: sharp, severe
egr*e* (1×)

elementt, *n*. One of the four simple substances, earth, water, air, and fire (to which a fifth, the ether, was sometimes added), of which all material bodies were assumed to be compounded
Elementt (1×)

elenacampana, *n*. Elecampane, horseheal
Elenaca*m*pana (2×)

emitriceus, *n*. A kind of intermittent fever
Emit*ri*ceus (1×), Emit*ri*ceu*m* (1×)

empima, *n*. Empyema, a disease characterised by a gathering of pus in the pleura
Empima (1×)

Empostym > **postym**, *n*.

emrawdys, *n*. Haemorrhoids, esp. the bleeding kind
Emrawdys (13×)

enchaffen, *v*. To make physically warm or hot; to warm, heat
Enchaffyng (1×)

enclosen, *v*. To close, shut
enclosyd (2×)

encorporacion, *n*. The act of combining of substances, blending (a sense that relates to how the ypostasis is or is not blended with the fluid part of the urine)
Encorp*or*acion (1×)

encorporaten, *v*. To blend
Encorp*or*at (1×)

ende, *n*. End; termination
ende (8×), end (1×)

enden, *v*. To stop, cease
ende (1×), endyth (1×)

endyng, *ng*. Ending, a coming to an end
endyng (1×)

endyve, *n*. A plant similar to wild lettuce, having small yellow flowers and seeds like a dandelion; perhaps sowthistle or corn sowthistle
Endyve (1×), yndyue (1×)

enfeccion, *n*. An infectious disease; any kind of disease
enfecc*i*on (1×)

enfecten, *v*. To infect
enfectyth (1×), enfecte (1×)

engendren, *v*. to beget or have (offspring); be begotten, born, or descended; produce, cause (something)
engendryd (6×), egendryd (1×), gendryd (1×)

entens, *adj*. Great, extreme, intense
entens (1×)

epiglotum, *n*. The epiglottis
Epiglotum (2×), Epiglotu*m* (1×)

epilencie, *n*. Epilepsy
Epilencie (2×), Epilencia (1×), Epilensye (1×)

equal, *adj*. Identical in amount, extent, or portion
equal (5×)

ere, *n*. The ear
Erys (3×)

erthe, *n*. Earth
erthe (1×)

ese, *n.* Relief from physical pain or suffering
ese (1×)

esily, *adv.* Easily
esily (1×), hesily (1×)

esy, *adj.* Calm, undisturbed
esy (1×)

et cetera, *n.* And so forth, and so on
&c (10×), &c. (1×)

eten, *v.* To eat
Ete (2×)

ethiopp, *n.* An inhabitant of Ethiopia
Ethiopp (1×)

ethymologies, *n.* A methodical discussion of the origins, or true meanings, of words; specif., Isidore of Seville's *Etymologiae* (*Etymologiarvm sive originvm Libri XX)*
Ethymologies (1×)

etyk, *n.* A continuous wasting fever
Etyk (2×)

etyk, *adj.* Suffering from hectic fever
Etyk (14×), etyck (1×), Etyk (1×)

etyng, *n.* The act or habit of eating
etyng (1×)

euenten, *v.* To let blood by cupping (cf. *aventen*)
euentyd (1×)

evyl, *n.* A disease, sickness
evyl (16×), euyl (1×)

evyn, *n.* Evening
evyn (3×), eue*n* (1×)

excesse > **accesse**, *n.*

excesse, *n.* Excess or excessiveness in number, amount, or quantity
excesse (11×), excesse (1×)

eye, *n.* Eye
Eyen (2×), eyes (1×)

eyre, *n.* Air
eyr*e* (1×)

F

face, *n.* The face
ffаce (4×), face (1×)

fallen, *v.* To descend, fall
fallyth (2×), fall (1×), falle (1×), fallyn (1×)

fallyng, *ng.* Falling, dropping; decreasing
ffallyng (2×)

fallyng evyl, *n.* Epilepsy
fallyng evyl (1×)

famose, *adj.* Foamy
ffamose (1×)

faren, *v.* To go, move away
faryth (1×)

fasten, *v.* To abstain voluntarily from food and drink
ffastyth (1×)

fastyng, *ng.* Voluntary abstinence from food and drink
ffastyng (1×)

fatnes, *n.* Fat, grease
fatnes (5×), ffatnes (4×), fattnes (1×), ffattnes (2×)

fatte, *adj.* Fat; thick, dense
ffatte (4×), fatt (2×), fatte (2×), ffatt (1×)

fatty, *adj.* Greasy, surfaced like fat
ffatty (8×), fatty (7×)

fattysh, *adj.* Greasy, oily
ffattysh (1×), ffattyssh (1×)

faylen, *v.* To prove unsuccessful; go wrong
ffayle (1×)

faylynge, *ng.* Lack of success, failure
faylyng (1×), ffaylyng (1×)

fayr, *adj.* Pure; clean
ffayr (2×), ffayr*e* (1×)

feblen, *v.* To become weak or infirm
ffeblyn (1×), ffeblyth (1×)

froth, *n*. Foam, spume, froth
ffroth (6×), froth (5×), ffroth (1×), frothys (1×)

frothy, *adj*. Foamy, frothy
ffrothy (1×)

fundmentte, *n*. The lower extremity of the rectum, the anus
fu*n*dmentte (1×)

ful, *adj*. Full
ffull (5×), fful (3×), full (2×), ffulle (1×), ful (1×)

fully, *adv*. Fully, completely
ffully (1×)

fume, *n*. Foam, spume, froth; smoke
ffume (5×), ffome (1×), fume (2×), fome (1×)

fumittere, *n*. Fumitory
ffumitt*erre* (1×)

furfura, *n*. Scales, scurf
furfura (2×), ffurfura (2×), ffurfurca (2×), ffurffura (1×), ffurphurijs (1×)

fuske, *adj*. Dark in colour, dusky
fuske (1×)

fylth, *n*. Filth
fylth (1×)

fynden, *v*. To find
ffowndyn (1×)

fynger, *n*. A finger
ffyngris (1×), ffyngrys (1×)

fynkell, *n*. Fennel
ffynkell (1×)

fynne, *adj*. Of supreme or select quality, choice; excellent
ffynne (1×)

fyre, *n*. Fire
fyr*e* (1×)

fysh, *n*. Fish
ffysshys (2×) ffych (1×), ffysh (1×), ffyssh (1×)

G

gaderen, *v*. To gather
gad*e*ren (1×), gaderyd (1×)

galle, *n*. The gall bladder of man or animal
galle (4×)

galon, *n*. A liquid measure of capacity, a gallon
galon (1×)

Galterius, *n*. Walter of Agilon, a French physician (c. 1250–1306)
Galt*eri*u*s* (14×), Galt*erium* (1×), Galt*erium* (1×), Galt*e*rius (1×), Galt*eriu*s (2×)

Galyen, *n*. Galen of Pergamon, the prominent Greek physician, surgeon and phylosopher in the Roman Empire (c. 130–c. 210)
Galyen (6×), Galien (2×), Galien*us* (2×), Galien*us* (2×), Gallyen (1×), Galyen (1×)

garlek, *n*. Garlic
garlek (1×)

garlon, *n*. A region of the urinal, a garland-like region near the top of the urine flask
garlon (1×)

gendren, *v*. To produce, bring forth, make
gend*er* (1×)

general, *adj*. Of wide application, generic, general
gen*e*ral (2×)

generatif, *adj*. Procreative, reproductive
gen*era*tivys (1×)

generatif, *n*. The generative members (a reproductive or excretory organ) including the kidneys and the bladder
gen*e*ratiues (1×), gen*era*ti*uis* (1×), gen*e*rativis (1×), gen*er*tiuys (1×), gene*ratiuis* (1×)

gete, *n.* A plant whose seeds were used as a condiment (Nigella sativa)
gete (1×)

Gilbertus, *n.* Gilbertus Anglicus, also known Gilbert of England or Gilbertinus, the English physician (c. 1180–c. 1250)
Gilber (2×), Gilbertum (1×), Gilbertum (2×), Gilbertum (1×), Gilbertus (2×), Gilbertus (2×), Gilbertus (16×), Gilbertus (1×), *Gilbertus* (1×)

gingre, *n.* Ginger
gingre (1×), gynger (1×), gyngre (1×)

gladly, *adv.* Readily, easily, freely
gladly (1×)

glasse, *n.* Glass
glasse (2×)

glauke, *adj.* Whitish yellow, yellow like a shining horn
Glauke (4×), glauca (3×), glauka (1×), glauke (1×), clauke (1×)

gleba, *n.* Soil, earth
gleba (1×), gleba (1×)

glet, *n.* Viscous or slimy animal matter; phlegm, mucus
glet (1×), glett (3×)

gleymouse, *adj.* Slimy, sticky, viscous
gleymouse (1×), gleymowse (1×)

gnawyng, *ng.* A tormenting pain; colic, pain in the gums or joints
gnawyng (2×)

gobet, *n.* A fragment
gobettis (2×)

God, *n.* God
god (2×)

gold, *n.* Gold
gold (2×)

golde, *n.* The European marigold
Goldys (1×)

gomor, *n.* Gonorrhoea
gomore (2×), gomorrea (1×), gomorrea (1×)

gon, *v.* To go
goyth (5×), goo (4×), goyng (2×), goon (2×), goyn (1×), went (1×), wentte (1×)

good, *adj.* Good
good (23×), better (4×), best (1×), beste (1×)

Gordianus, *n.* Bernard de Gordon, a French doctor and professor of medicine (1270–1330)
Gordianus (35×), Gordianus (3×), Gordianum (2×), Gordyanus (2×), Gordianus (1×), Gordianus (1×)

goutte, *n.* An attack of gout; a painful swelling; an arthritic swelling
goutte (8×), goutis (1×), gouttis (1×), gowtte (1×)

gowtus, *adj.* Inducing the gout
gowtus (1×)

grace, *n.* God's grace
grace (1×)

grainy, *adj.* Like grain, lumpy, spotted with pustules
grayny (1×)

granulosa, *adj.* Grainy, lumpy
granulosa (1×)

grauel, *n.* Sand
grauel (12×), grauel (1×), gravel (1×)

grauely, *adj.* Sandy, covered with gravel or sand; containing calculous matter resembling sand
grauely (1×)

grece, *n.* The fat of an animal
grece (1×), grece (1×), grose (1×)

grecynesse, *n.* Greasiness, oiliness
grecynesse (1×)

greffe, *n.* Sickness, disease, bodily defect or injury
greffe (1×)

Grek, *n.* Greece
grek (1×)
grene, *adj.* The colour green
grene (30×), g*re*ne (4×), gre*n* (1×)
grenesse, *n.* Green colour
grenesse (4×), g*re*nes (1×), g*re*nesse (1×)
grenysh, *adj.* Somewhat green, dull or pale green
grenysh (3×), g*re*nysh (3×), grenyssh (1×)
gresse, *n.* Grass
gresse (1×)
grete, *adj.* Large in size or quantity, big; great
grete (42×), g*re*te (22×), g*re*tt*er* (4×), grett (2×), greet (1×)
gretly, *adv.* Earnestly, strongly, heartily
gretly (1×)
greuaunce, *n.* Sickness, disease
greuau*n*ce (1×), g*re*uau*n*ce (1×), grevance (1×)
greven, *v.* To cause physical injury; wound, damage
g*re*vyd (3×), g*re*uyd (2×)
grey, *adj.* Ash-coloured, dull, grey
grey (1×)
greyn, *n.* Seed, grain; Something resembling grain
greynes (5×), g*re*nys (3×), grana (1×), g*ra*nula (1×), granu*m* (1×), g*ra*nys (1×), grenes (1×), greynys (1×)
greynes, *n.* Grayness, grey colour
greynes (4×), greynys (2×)
gromyle, *n.* The common gromwell
g*ro*myle (2×)
grose, *n.* Sediment; the thick part of a humour; the large section of a bodily part or organ
g*ro*se (1×)
grose, *adj.* Thick, heavy
g*ro*se (13×), grose (5×), gross (1×), grosse (1×)
grownde, *n.* The lowest part (of a liquid)
grownde (2×), g*ro*wnde (2×), g*ro*unde (1×), grow*n*d (1×), grow*n*de (1×)
Gru, *n.* The Greek language
gru (1×)
gut, *n.* The human intestines
gut (1×), gutt*is* (5×), guttys (2×)
gutta, *n.* ~ rosacea, pustules on the face or body
Gutta (1×)
Gyles, *n.* Giles de Corbeil, a French royal physician (c. 1140–1224)
gyles (1×)

H

hakyng > **akyng**, *ng.*
halff, *n.* Half; a quantity, a unit of measurement
halff (1×), halffe (1×)
hand, *n.* Hand
hand (2×), handys (1×), handys (1×), honde (1×), hondys (1×)
handful, *n.* A handful
handfful (1×)
hangen, *v.* To hang, suspend
hangyth (2×), hang (1×), hangyng (1×), hangy*n*g (1×)
hard, *adj.* Hard, difficult, troublesome
hard (3×), harde (1×)
hardnes, *n.* Physical hardness
hardnes (1×), hardenes (1×)
hasty, *adj.* Swift, quick
hasty (3×)
haunch, *n.* The hips, haunch
haunch (1×), hau*n*che (1×)
haven, *v.* To have
haue (33×), haþ (15×), hayth (8×), hayþ (7×), hath (6×), havyng (3×), had (2×),

han (2×), haþe (1×), haue (1×), [haue] (1×), hauy*ng* (1×)

hawntyng, *ng.* The act of frequenting a place
hawntyng (1×)

hed, *n.* Head
hed (35×), hede (1×)

hedach, *n.* Hedache
hedach (1×)

helen, *v.* To cure, heal
hele (2×)

helpe, *n.* Help, assistance
helpe (1×)

helpen, *v.* To help
holpe (1×)

helthe, *n.* Health
helthe (6×), helth (3×), onhelthe (1×)

henbane, *n.* Henbane
henbane (1×)

her, *n.* Hair
herys (5×), heer*e* (2×), heir (1×), heir*e* (1×), heyr*e* (1×)

herb, *n.* Herb
h*er*b*is* (1×)

herbe benet, *n.* One of two plants used for medicine: the common hemlock or the common avens
h*er*be benet (3×)

hereof, *adv.* From this place, from here
her*e*of (1×)

herte, *n.* Heart
herte (4×), h*er*te (9×)

hertistung, *n.* The hart's-tongue fern
h*er*t*is*tung (1×), hertystu*ng* (1×)

hervest, *n.* The season of autumn, fall
hervest (2×), heruest (1×)

hesily > **esily**, *b.*

hete, *n.* Heat; high body temperature caused by sickness or fever
hete (29×), hetis (1×)

hevy, *adj.* Heavy
hevy (1×)

hevynesse, *n.* Physical heaviness, weight
hevynesse (3×), hevynes (1×)

hey, *adj.* Intense, deep (of colour)
hey (1×)

hiȝe, *adj.* High, big, tall
hiȝe (1×), hiþ*er* (1×), hiȝ (1×), hiȝer (1×), hiȝest (1×), hyȝe (1×), hiyer (1×)

hoge, *adj.* Great, powerful
hoge (1×)

hold > **olde**, *a.*

holden, *v.* To keep, retain, hold
hold (1×), holde (1×), holdyng (1×)

holdyng, *ng.* The action of grasping, grip
holdyng (1×)

holounesse, *n.* The small of the back
holounesse (1×)

holpe > **helpen**, *v.*

hony, *n.* Honey
hony (5×)

hool, *adj.* Healthy, cured
hool (4×), hooll (2×), hole (1×), holl (1×)

hope, *n.* Hope
hope (4×)

horehound, *n.* The common herb horehound
hor*e*hound (2×), horehounde (1×)

horn, *n.* A horn of cattle, sheep, goats, etc.
horn (1×), horne (1×)

horse, *n.* A horse
horse (1×)

hote, *adj.* Hot
hote (16×), hott (1×), hott*er* (1×)

hote feuer, *n.* The feverish stage of ague; violent fever
hote feu*er* (1×)

house, *n.* A house
house (1×)

L

labour, *n.* Work, hard work
labo*ur* (2×)
lacteus, *adj.* White as whey
lacte*us* (5×), lactea (2×), lacte*us* (1×), lacteus (1×)
lakkyng, *ng.* A lack, absence
lakkyng (1×)
lanke > **flanke**, *n.*
lapis, *n.* Kidney and bladder stones
lapis (1×)
large, *adj.* Ample in quantity; abundant, copious
large (1×)
largenesse, *n.* Great size; width
largenesse (1×)
last, *adj.* Last
last (2×), laste (2×)
lasten, *v.* To last
laste (2×), lastyd (1×), lastyng (1×), lastyþ (1×), lastyth (1×)
late, *adv.* Late
late (2×)
Laten, *n.* The Latin language
laten (1×)
leche, *n.* A bloodsucking worm
leche (2×)
lechery, *n.* Lechery
lechery (3×)
led, *n.* Lead
led (1×)
ledere, *n.* Leather
leder*e* (1×)
ledy, *adj.* Lead-coloured, dull
ledy (7×)
ledysh, *adj.* Lead-coloured, dull
ledysh (4×)
leen, *adj.* Lean, slender; thin from disease
leen (1×), lene (1×)
leennes, *n.* Leanness, thinness
lee*n*nes (1×), leennesse (1×)
lef, *n.* A leaf
levys (1×)
leffte, *adj.* Left
leffte (3×), leffte (1×), lyffte (1×)
leg, *n.* The human leg
legg*is* (2×), leggys (1×)
leien, *v.* To put, place, set
ley (3×), leyd (1×)
lek, *n.* A leek
lek*is* (1×)
lendes, *n.* The human loins
lendys (5×)
lesen, *v.* To lessen
lesen (1×), lose (1×)
lesse, *adj.* Less; least
lesse (6×), lest (1×)
leten, *v.* To let; allow, grant
leet (1×), let (2×), lett (1×)
letten, *v.* To hinder, impede, delay
lettyd (2×)
leucofflewma, *n.* Leucophlegmasia, lymphatic edema
leucofflewma (1×), leucofflewma (1×)
liȝt, *adj.* Light; free of pain; relieved of an illness
liȝtt (4×), lyȝtt (2×), liȝtte (1×), liȝtt*er* (1×), lyȝhtt (1×), lyȝt (1×)
liȝtnes, *n.* Brightness
liȝtnes (1×)
liȝtsom, *adj.* Relieved from disease
lyȝtsom (1×)
litiasy, *n.* Kidney stone
litiasy (1×)
liuidus, *adj.* Of a bluish leaden colour, livid
liuid*us* (10×), livid*us* (5×), lyuyd*us* (2×), liuid*us* (1×), liuyde (1×), lividi (1×), livid*us* (1×), livyde (1×)
loken, *v.* To look
loke (3×)
long, *adj.* Long-lasting, long
long (26×), leng*er* (1×)

long, *adv.* For a long time, long
long (1×)

longen, *v.* To belong
long (1×)

losenyng, *ng.* Loosening (of the bowels)
losenyng (1×)

loth, *adj.* Hateful, unpleasant
loth (1×)

louh, *adj.* Low, inferior
louh (6×), lowh (4×), louhwer*e* (1×), louhȝ (1×), lowere (1×),

lumppy, *adj.* In one piece, in a lump or clump (at the bottom of the urinal)
lu*m*ppy (1×)

lumpyng, *adj.* Lumpish, heavy
lu*m*pyng (1×)

lunge, *n.* The human or animal lung
lu*n*g*is* (7×), lu*n*gg*is* (5×), lu*n*ggis (1×), lungg*is* (1×), lung*is* (1×), lungys (1×)

luste, *n.* Desire, wish, will
luste (1×)

lusten, *v.* To wish, desire; take pleasure, like
lustyth (1×)

lych, *adj.* Like
lych (1×)

lycorys, *n.* The dried root of the plant Glycyrrhiza glabra, used in medicine and cooking; liquorice; the plant itself
lycorys (1×), licoryis (1×), lycoriys (1×)

lyff, *n.* Life, lifetime
lyff (6×), lyffe (2×), lyfe (1×)

lykenen, *v.* To compare
lykeyn (1×)

lyking, *ng.* A feeling or experience of pleasure, enjoyment
lyking (1×), lykyng (1×)

lym, *n.* A member of the body
ly*m*mys (1×)

lynnen, *adj.* Consisting of linen
ly*n*nen (1×)

lynsed, *n.* The seed of flax, linseed
lynsed (1×)

lyppotomia, *n.* Fainting, swooning
lyppotomia (1×)

lytel, *adj.* Little, not much
lytel (28×), litel (10×), lytell (5×), litell (2×), liȝtt (1×), lytyl (1×)

lyven, *v.* To live
lyve (1×)

lyver, *n.* The human liver
lyu*er* (51×), lyuer (2×), <u>lyuer</u> (1×)

lyuerwort, *n.* The common liverwort
lyu*er*wortt (2×), lyu*er*wort (1×)

M

maken, *v.* To make, prepare; produce
make (8×), made (4×), makyng (1×), makyth (1×)

maledy, *n.* A disease; sickness
maledyes (3×), maledy (11×),

malencoly, *n.* A disease, sickness; one of the four humours, black bile
malencoly (20×), <u>Malencoly</u> (6×), male*n*coly (4×), male*n*coli (1×), malencoli (1×), malencolica*m* (1×), m*elancol*iam (1×), m*e*la*ncolia*ȝ (1×)

malencolyk, *adj.* Having a pathological condition of the black bile
malencolyk (1×)

malice, *n.* Harmful or dangerous quality; poor quality
malice (1×)

malicious, *adj.* Poisonous, malignant
malicious (1×)

man, *n.* A person, a man or woman
man (11×), men (7×), ma*n*nys (6×), ma*n* (2×)

maner, *n.* Type, kind, sort
man*er* (24×), maner*e* (1×)

mansuron, *n.* Probably denoting either blindness (*no poure of seyng*) or strangury (Gr. mans + οὖρον)
mansuron (1×)

marubium, *n.* The common or white horehound
marubiu*m* (1×)

mastyk, *n.* Mastic, the resin exuded from the mastic tree
mastyk (1×)

mater, *n.* A bodily fluid; nutritive or humoral fluid in the venous blood
mat*er* (18×), mater (1×)

matfelon, *n.* Knapweed, matfellon
matfelon (1×), matfelo*u*n (1×)

matrice, *n.* The uterus, womb
mat*ri*ce (13×), mat*ri*ce (2×), matrice (1×), mat*ri*cis (1×), Mat*ri*x (1×)

maystren, *v.* To prevail, predominate; reduce
mayst*ri* (1×)

maystri, *n.* Predominance of one element, humour, or accidental circumstance in a mixture or complexion; dominance
mayst*ri* (1×), mast*ri* (1×)

medicyn, *n.* A medicine, medicament
medicyn (1×)

medlen, *v.* To blend, mix
medlyd (2×), medyl (2×), medle (1×)

mele, *n.* Meal made by grinding grain; flour
mele (2×)

meltyng, *ng.* Melting; liquefaction
meltyng (3×)

membre, *n.* A bodily limb or organ
me*m*bris (16×), me*m*brys (11×), me*m*b*er* (7×), membrys (2×), me*m*br*a* (1×), membr*a* (1×), membris (1×), me*m*br*is* (1×), me*m*bror*um* (1×), me*m*brys (1×)

mene, *adj.* Of a mixed quality or character
mene (5×)

menely, *adv.* With moderation, moderately
menely (12×), menly (1×)

mengen, *v.* To mix, mingle, blend
meyntt (2×), megtt (1×), mengyd (1×), menktt (1×), mey*n*gtt (1×), mentt (1×)

mercurye, *n.* The plant mercury
m*er*curye (1×)

mesure, *n.* Moderation in food, drink
mesur*e* (1×)

mete, *n.* Food, nourishment
met*is* (7×), mete (4×), metys (1×)

meten, *v.* To encounter, experience
mett (1×)

meven, *v.* To move
mevyng (1×)

mid, *n.* The middle, middle part of something
myddys (1×)

miȝt, *n.* Ability, capacity; a skill, knowledge
myȝtt (1×), myȝtt*is* (1×)

miȝty, *adj.* Mighty
myȝty (1×)

milke, *n.* Milk
mylke (2×)

milky, *adj.* Milk-white, milky
mylky (3×), Milky (2×)

mirabolan indicum, *n.* Indian mirabolans, the fruit of several species of Terminalia, used medicinally
mirabolan Iudicu*m* (1×)

mirabolanorum, *n.* The fruit of several species of Terminalia, used medicinally
mirabolanor*um* (1×)
miscen, *v.* To mix, blend
misc*e* (1×)
moch, *adv.* Much, greatly
moch (2×), moche (1×)
mocyon, *n.* Motion
mocyon (1×)
moddy, *adj.* Muddy
moddy (1×), mody (1×)
modyr, *n.* The uterus of a woman, womb
modyr (1×)
moleyne, *n.* The herb mullein
moleyne (1×), moleyn (1×)
month, *n.* A calendar month
month (2×), monthys (1×)
morfu, *n.* A skin disease characterised by leprous or scurfy eruptions, morphea
morffu (1×)
morowe, *n.* Morning, dawn, break of day
morowe (1×)
morter, *n.* A mortar, a bowl used for grinding and mixing ingredients
mort*er* (1×)
mortifycacion, *n.* Destruction of natural heat (through excessive cold)
mortifycac*i*on (6×), mortificac*i*on (3×), Mortificac*i*on (2×), mortyfycac*i*on (2×), mortifycacio*u*n (2×), mortific*i*on (1×), mortifycacio*u*n (1×), Mortyficac*i*on (1×)
morwe, *n.* Morning, the early part of the day
morwe (1×)
moste, *adv.* Most, in the highest degree
moste (14×), most (6×), moost (1×)
mot, *n.* A speck, particle, bit of dirt or foreign matter; an impurity in drink
mot*is* (2×), motis (1×), motys (3×)
moten, *v.* To be allowed, be permitted, may
must (1×), muste (1×)
movyng, *ng.* Moving, motion; a movement
movyng (1×)
mowen, *v.* May; be able, be capable
may (11×), mayst (3×), mow (1×)
mowth, *n.* The human mouth
mowth (3×), mowthe (2×)
moyste, *adj.* Moist, wet
moyste (1×), moyst (1×)
moyste, *n.* The quality of moistness
moyste (1×)
moystnesse, *n.* Moisture, wetness
moystnesse (3×), moystnes (2×)
moystoure, *n.* Moisture, wetness
moystour*e* (2×), moysted (1×)
multitud, *n.* A large amount, abundance; mass
multitud (1×), multytud (1×)
mustela, *n.* A weasel
mustela (1×)
mydel, *n.* The middle part of a thing
mydel (5×)
myddys, *n.* The middle part of something, midst
myddys (8×), myddis (2×), mydys (1×)
mydryff, *n.* The diaphragm of man or animal
mydryff (9×), mydr*i*ff (1×)
mykel, *adj.* In a large amount, much
mykel (4×), mykyl (2×)
mykyl, *adv.* Much, greatly; deeply
mykyl (1×)
mylffoyle, *n.* Milfoil, yarrow
mylffoyle (1×)

oyle, *n.* A specific oil
oyle (7×)

oyly, *adj.* Resembling oil, oily
oyly (5×)

oylysh, *adj.* Oilish, resembling oil
oylysh (3×), oylish (1×)

oynment, *n.* An ointment, medicinal salve for external application
oy*n*ment (1×), oy*n*me*n*tt*is* (1×)

P

pacyent, *n.* Patient, person under medical supervision
pacyent (6×), pacient (1×), pacyentte (1×)

pale, *adj.* Light, pale, as it were the broth of flesh that is half sodden[6]
pale (24×), pale (2×)

palsy, *n.* The failure of a part of the body to function properly; loss of motor power, paralysis; loss of tactile sensation; numbness
palsy (2×), palsy (1×), palsye (1×)

palysh, *adj.* Somewhat pale or pallid
palysh (1×)

pantegni, *n.* The Pantegni book, Constantine's translation of Haly Abba's *Liber Regalis/Kitab al-Malaki*, the first major Arabic text to be translated into Latin and one of the major sources of the Latin tradition of medicine as a compendium of Hellenistic and Islamic medicine (c. 1086)[7]
pan*tegni* (1×), panteg*n*i (1×), pantegni (1×)

pappe, *n.* A woman's breast
pappis (1×), pappys (1×)

parbraken, *v.* To vomit
p*ar*brakyng (1×), parbrakyth (1×)

[6] Taken from Stolberg (2015: 35).

[7] See (French 2003: 85) for a full account of the different translations of the Pantegni book.

parbrakyng, *ng.* Vomiting
p*ar*brakyng (1×), p*ar*bragyng (1×)

part, *n.* A part of a whole, portion
p*ar*t (6×), p*ar*ty (6×), partyes (2×), p*ar*tyes (2×), Partes (1×), p*ar*tes (1×), p*ar*ties (1×), p*ar*tiys (1×)

passen, *v.* To exceed, surpass; move, advance
passyng (5×), passyth (2×)

passio, *n.* An ailment, a disease, an attack of fever
passio (7×), passion (3×), pasio (1×), passio (1×), passyo (1×), passyon (1×)

passyng, *ng.* Going by, passing
passyng (1×)

peleter, *n.* Common pellitory, pellitory of the wall
pelet*er* (1×)

penawnce, *n.* Pain, suffering
penawnce (2×), penavnce (1×)

pentaloyde, *n.* Husks of grain, flake-like partioculates between *furfura* and *crinoides*
pentoloyde (1×), pentaloides (1×)

peper, *n.* The dried berries of the pepper plant
pep*er* (1×)

perceyven, *v.* To perceive; hear, feel, taste, or smell
p*er*ceyvyd (1×)

perdycion, *n.* Great harm; death
p*er*dyc*i*on (1×)

pere, *n.* A pear
pere (1×)

perel, *n.* Peril, danger
perel (13×), perell (2×)

perfecte, *adj.* Complete
perfecte (1×)

perforat, *adj.* Perforated, pierced
perforat (1×)

peripleumonia, *n.* An inflammation of the lungs; pneumonia
peripleumonia (2×), perileumonia (1×), perilpleumonia (1×), peripleumonia (1×), peripleumonia (1×)

perlous, *adj.* Dangerous
perlous (1×)

persly, *n.* Parsley
persly (5×)

persone, *n.* An individual, a person
persone (1×)

peryn > **aperen**, *v.*

pestylence, *n.* An infectious or contagious disease; a fatal epidemic or disease, plague
pestylence (2×), pestilence (1×), pestilence (1×)

peyne, *n.* Physical pain
peyne (62×), peyne (1×)

pinguis, *adj.* Fat, thick
pinguis (1×), pinguis (1×)

pisse, *n.* Urine
pisse (1×), pysse (1×)

place, *n.* Place, locality, spot
place (5×), placis (2×), plac*is* (2×), placys (2×), place (1×)

plaster, *n.* A plaster, poultice, or compress made from herbs, meal, or other substance
plast*er* (3×)

plente, *n.* Abundance
plente (4×)

plot, *n.* Ypostasis in the urinal, when it appears in separated pieces
plottys (1×)

pluresis, *n.* Pleurisy, inflammation of the membrane surrounding the lungs and lining the thoracic cavity
pluresis (5×), pluresys (2×), plueresis (1×), plurecis (1×), pluresis (1×), pluresis (1×), pluresy (1×)

polipody, *n.* The common polypody
polipody (1×)

polucyon, *n.* Discharge of semen other than during sexual intercourse
polucyon (1×)

popilyon, *n.* An ointment in which poplar leaves or buds are the principal ingredient
popilyon (1×)

popy, *n.* Opium poppy or any of the varieties of this plant
popy (1×)

porcyon, *n.* A portion or segment of something
porcyon (1×)

pore, *n.* Power, ability
por*e* (1×)

porette, *n.* A thick soup made with chickpeas, onions, etc.
porrett*is* (1×)

porke, *n.* The flesh of swine used for food, pork
porke (1×)

pose, *n.* A head cold; catarrh
pose (1×)

postym, *n.* Any morbid swelling or inflammation in any part of the body
postym (19×), postem (6×), empostyms (2×), Empostemmys (1×), Empostym (1×)

potage, *n.* A thick soup or stew, variously with or without meat
potage (2×), patage (1×)

potager, *n.* Gout in the foot, podagra
Potag*er* (1×)

potel, *n.* A vessel of half the capacity of the associated gallon measure; a pottle
potel (1×)

pounce, *n.* A stab, thrust
pounce (1×)

poure, *n.* Efficacy; power
pour*e* (1×), power*e* (1×)

pouryng, *ng.* The pouring on of water
pouryng (1×)

powder, *n.* Powder; a medicinal powder used in preparing ointments or potions
powd*er* (5×), poud*er* (3×)

poynte, *n.* A subject, topic, theme
poyntis (1×)

prassina, *adj.* Leek-green
prassina (1×)

precipitacion, *n.* The separation of a solid substance from a solution, precipitation
p*re*cipitac*i*o*n* (2×), p*re*cipitac*i*o*n* (1×), p*re*cipitac*i*o*n*is (1×)

principal, *adj.* Main, principal, dominant
p*ri*ncipal (1×)

principaly, *adv.* Mostly, mainly, primarily
p*ri*ncipaly (2×), p*ri*ncipali (1×), p*ri*ncipally (1×)

privy, *adj.* Private, personal
p*ri*vy (1×)

prolongacioun, *n.* Delay, postponement
prolongacio*u*n (1×), p*ro*longacio*u*n (1×)

propyr, *adj.* Correct, appropriate, proper
p*ro*pyr (1×)

pryckyng, *ng.* Smarting, sharp pain; prickling, irritation
pryckyng (4×), p*ri*ckyng (2×), prytchyng (1×)

pure, *adj.* Pure, uncontaminated
pur*e* (4×), pure (2×)

purgacion, *n.* The evacuation of evil humours through the use of cathartics, emetics, or bloodletting
p*ur*gacion (1×), p*ur*gac*i*on (1×)

purgen, *v.* To cleanse, purge by a laxative, a diuretic, or an emetic
p*ur*ge (1×)

purpyl, *adj.* Purple, dark crimson, violet
p*ur*pyl (3×)

puryfien, *v.* To cleanse, clarify, clean
puryfied (1×)

pus, *n.* Pus, matter
pus (1×)

push, *n.* A pustule, pimple, boil
pusshys (1×)

putredo, *n.* A state of putrefaction, festering; gangrene; pus, suppurating matter
put*re*do (2×)

putredus, *adj.* Putrid
put*re*d*us* (1×)

putrifien, *v.* To decompose, rot
put*ri*fied (1×)

putten, *v.* To put, apply
put (7×)

puttyng, *ng.* Expulsion, eviction
puttyng (1×)

pyckyng, *ng.* Plucking (at)
pyckyng (1×)

pylliol mowntein, *n.* Wild thyme; pennyroyal
pylliol mownteyn (1×)

pyneappyl, *n.* A pine cone
pyneappyl (1×)

pynguedo, *n.* Grease
pynguedo (1×)

pyony, *n.* Peony
pyony (1×)

pype, *n.* A tube, duct or vessel of the human body; the urethra of the male
pypis (2×), pipys (1×)

pyssen, *v.* To piss, urinate
pyssyd (3×), pisse (2×), pysse (1×)

pyssyng, *ng.* The act of urinating
pyssyng (2×)

Q

quaken, *v.* To shake because of illness or a physical infirmity, a wound, etc.
quake (1×), q*ua*kyth (1×)

quakyng, *ng.* Trembling, quivering, or shivering because of illness or other physical cause
quakyng (1×)

quantyte, *n.* Quantity, amount
qua*n*tyte (10×), qu*an*tyte (9×), quantyte (8×), qu*an*tite (2×), qua*n*tite (2×)

quart, *n.* A liquid measure of capacity, a quart
quart (1×)

quarteyn, *n.* Quartan fever
quarteyn (2×), q*ua*rteyn (1×), quarteyns (1×)

quarteyn, *adj.* Quartan (fever)
quarteyn (1×)

quaveren, *v.* To quake, waver
quav*er*yt (1×)

quenchen, *v.* To extinguish
que*n*chyd (1×), que*n*chyng (1×)

quyttur, *n.* Pus, suppuration
quytt*ur* (2×), quitt*er* (1×), quyt*er* (1×), quytt*er* (1×)

R

radical, *adj.* Vital or fundamental to life
radical (1×)

ragge, *n.* A shred of putrid matter in an ulcerated wound
Ragg*is* (1×)

Rasus, *n.* Rhazes the physician (865–925)
Ras*us* (1×)

raw, *adj.* Uncooked; undigested, unadapted; injured, lacerated, skinned, bloody
raw (7×), rawe (3×)

rauyn, *n.* The raven; the carrion crow
rauy*n*nys (1×)

ravyng, *n.* Delirium, mental derangement
ravyng (4×)

recipe, *n.* Recipe
R*ecipe* (1×)

recure, *n.* Recovery or relief from illness, distress
recur*e* (1×)

red, *adj.* The colour red
red (57×), red (2×), rede (1×)

redy, *adj.* Prepared, ready
redy (2×)

redysh, *adj.* Somewhat red, having a red tinge
redysh (2×)

rednesse, *n.* The state or quality of being red, redness
rednesse (2×), rednes (2×)

region, *n.* A part of the body; a division of a vessel of urine
region (14×), Regiouns (2×), region (1×), regiones (1×), regio*un* (1×), Regioun (1×)

reersen, *v.* To narrate, report, tell
reersyd (2×)

reyne, *n.* A human or an animal kidney
reynes (50×), reynes (3×), Renes (2×), reynys (1×)

remyshnes, *n.* The condition of being less intense, dull, dim (not as a result of dilution)
remyshnes (1×)

rennen, *v.* To flow
re*n*ne (1×)

rennyng, *ng.* Running
re*n*ny*ng* (1×), rennyng (1×)

replecion, *n.* Eating or drinking to excess
replecion (1×)

resolucion, *n.* A precipitate, sediment; the dispersal of an infection, a morbid humour
resoluc*i*ons (11×), resolucions (2×), resoluc*ions* (2×), resolucio*u*ns (1×), resolucyo*u*ns (1×)

reste, *n.* Rest
reste (1×), reste (1×), rest (1×)

resten, *v.* To take repose
restyd (1×)

restẏng, *ng.* Resting, lying down
restyng (1×)

resydence, *n.* The sediment or ypostasis that settles to the bottom of the urinal
resydence (7×), resydens (2×), resyde*n*ce (1×)

resydent, *adj.* Dwelling, resident
resydent (2×)

retencion, *n.* The retention within the body of blood, esp. menstrual blood
retenc*i*on (4×), rete*n*cion (2×), Retenc*ion* (1×), retencion (1×), Retencio*u*n (1×), Retencyo*o*n (1×)

reule, *n.* A general principle, rule
Reule (2×), rewle (1×)

rewmatyk, *adj.* Of the nature of rheum; consisting of rheum
rewmatyk (1×), rewmatyck (1×), rematyk (1×),

rewme, *n.* A watery fluid or humour conceived as draining from the higher parts of the body, and capable of causing diseases; a secretion, flux; a cold in the head; catarrh
rewme (7×), rewm (1×)

ribbe, *n.* A human rib
rybbis (1×), rybbys (1×)

reggebon, *n.* The human spine
reggebon (1×)

ryȝtt, *adj.* Right, as opposed to left
ryȝtt (8×), ryȝt (6×), riȝt (5×), riȝtt (3×), Ryȝht (2×), riȝtte (1×), Ryht (1×), Ryȝtte (1×)

rysen, *v.* To move upward, ascend
rysyng (6×)

rysyng, *ng.* The act of rising, ascending
rysyng (2×), Rysi*ng* (1×), Rysy*ng* (1×)

rody, *adj.* Reddish, red; reddish yellow
rody (1×)

roffe, *n.* The roof of the mouth, palate
roffe (1×)

ropen, *v.* To become viscous
ropyng (1×)

roryng, *ng.* Growling of the stomach
roryng (1×)

rosacea, *adj.* Pustules on the face or body
rosacea (1×)

rose, *n.* A plant of the genus Rosa; the flower of this plant
rose (2×)

rosen, *adj.* Made of or consisting of roses
rosen (1×)

rosten, *v.* To roast
roste (1×)

rote, *n.* A root of a tree
rot*is* (3×), rotys (3×)

roten, *v.* To become putrid, decay
rotyd (1×), rotyng (1×), rotyth (1×)

rothed, *n.* Rottenness, putrefaction
Rothed (2×)

rott, *adj.* Spoiled, rotten
Rott (1×)

rotyn, *adj.* Rotten, putrid, festering || ~ blod, menstrual blood
rotyn (2×), rottyn (1×), roten (1×)

rownd, *adj.* Spherical in shape, circular
rownd (3×), rownde (3×)

rubarbe, *n.* Rhubarb
rubarbe (1×)

rubea, *adj.* Of a yellowish-orange colour (mostly like saffron)
Rubea (4×), rube*us* (3×), *su*brube*us* (1×)

rubicund, *adj.* Of the colour of fire or a flame
Rubicu*nd* (1×), Rubicu*n*da (1×), Rubicu*n*di (1×), rubicu*n*d*us* (1×)

rue, *n.* A plant of the genus Ruta, esp. common rue
Rue (1×)

ruffe, *adj.* Red, reddish, as red gold[8]
ruffe (7×), <u>Ruffe</u> (7×), Rufe (1×), <u>rufe</u> (1×), Ruffa (1×)

rupten, *v.* To break open
rupt (1×)

rust, *n.* Rust on iron or other metals
Rust (1×)

S

sad, *adj.* Solid (of bodily organs or members)
sad (1×)

sadnes, *n.* Solidness; firmness, solidity, hardness
sadnes (1×)

saferen, *v.* To smell; taste
saferyth (1×)

saferon, *n.* The saffron crocus (Crocus sativus)
saferon (1×), safferon (1×)

salt, *adj.* Salty || ~ fleume, salt phlegm; a skin ailment
salt (5×), saltt (1×)

saltnes, *n.* Saltiness
saltnes (1×)

same, *adj.* Identical; equal, same
same (3×)

sandaly, *n.* Sandalwood
sandaly (1×)

sangueyn, *adj.* Of a blood-red colour; caused by an excess of the humour blood
sangueyn (2×)

sanyes, *n.* Pus, a purulent discharge
Sanyes (6×), sanies (1×)

satirion, *n.* A name for the various kinds of orchid
satirion (2×)

sauour, *n.* Savour, taste
sauo*ur* (10×), savour (1×)

saveyn, *n.* The plant Juniperus sabina, often used medicinally
Saveyn (1×)

sawflewme, *n.* A skin ailment symptomatic of a type of leprosy originating in a humoral disorder, caused by sexual and dietary excess and characterised by red and black discolouration, pustules, swelling, loss of hair, etc.
sawfflewme (1×)

sawge, *n.* The herb sage
sawge (3×), sauge (2×)

saxiffrage, *n.* A plant of the genus Saxifraga, used medicinally
saxiffrage (1×)

[8] Taken from Stolberg (2015: 35).

scabbe, *n.* Any eruption on the skin, a pimple, a blotch, or eczema
scabbe (4×), scabbis (1×), scabys (1×)
scaby, *adj.* Scabby, rough, scurfy
scaby (1×)
scabyose, *n.* Any of the plants of the genus Scabiosa
Scabyose (1×)
scaldyng, *ng.* Inflammation, overheating (of a bodily organ)
scaldyng (4×), skaldyng (1×)
scale, *n.* Scales
scalis (3×), scalys (2×), scal*is* (1×)
scaly, *adj.* Scaly
scaly (1×)
scamonye, *n.* The root of scammony, or a gum resin obtained therefrom, used in purgative medicines
Scamonye (1×)
scapyng, *ng.* Avoiding of peril, trouble, escape from
Scapyng (1×)
schysel > **chysel**, *n.*
sciatica, *n.* The disease sciatica
Sciatica (1×)
scom, *n.* Froth, foam
scom (3×), scom (1×)
scotomia, *n.* Dizziness and dimness of sight
scotomia (1×)
scurffe, *n.* A scaly or scabby disease of the skin
scurffe (1×)
scyatica passio, *n.* The disease sciatica; of an inflammation: affecting the sciatic nerve
scyatica passio (1×)
sed, *n.* A seed; semen, sperm; the grain or ovule of a plant by which a new plant is propagated
sed (7×), seed (4×)
sedymen, *n.* Sediment
sedymen (5×), Sedymen (1×)
sege, *n.* A chamber pot, stool || gon to ~, to go to stool, void the bowels or bladder
sege (1×)
sen, *v.* To see
se (3×)
sene, *n.* The powdered leaves or pods of senna, a plant of the genus Cassia, esp. the Alexandrian senna or Tinnevelly senna
sene (2×), senuys (1×), cene (1×)
senue, *n.* Sinew, a fibrous cord connecting a muscle to a bone or other bodily part, a tendon; a muscle
senuys (6×)
separaten, *v.* To remove; to divide, keep apart
sep*ar*att (1×)
sethen, *v.* To boil, seethe
sethe (4×), sodyn (2×), soden (1×)
setwale, *n.* The root of a plant of the species Curcuma, esp. the long zedoary
setwale (1×)
sew, *n.* Broth
sewys (1×)
seyen, *v.* To say
seyth (9×), sey (3×), seyn (2×), seyst (2×), seyd (1×)
seyng, *n.* The act of seeing
seyng (1×)
shadwen, *v.* To provide shade
shadwyd (2×)
shadwyd, *adj.* Shaded, shadowy
shadwyd (2×)
shaken, *v.* To shake
shake (2×), shakyng (1×)
shappe, *n.* Form, shape
shappe (1×), shappe (1×)
share, *n.* The pubic region, groin
shar*e* (4×)
sharpe, *adj.* Acute, intense, severe || ~ feuer, acute, intense fever
sharpe (3×)

sharpnes, *n*. Sharp pain, painfulness
sharpnes (1×)

sheden, *v*. To pour
shedd (1×)

shedyng, *ng*. Spilling, dropping
shedyng (2×)

shete, *n*. A bed sheet
shet*is* (1×)

shetyng, *ng*. Causing affliction
shetyng (1×)

shewen, *v*. To show
shewyth (4×), shew*yth* (3×), shew (3×), shewe (2×), shewhyth (1×), shew*n* (1×), shewyd (1×), shewyþ (1×)

short, *adj*. Short (of breath), laboured, difficult
short (1×), shorte (1×), shortt (1×), shortte (1×), shrot (1×)

short, *adv*. With severe restriction, straitly, narrowly
short (1×)

shortnes, *n*. Difficulty (of breath), breathlessness, difficuklty in breathing, dyspnea
shortnes (1×)

shortwyndyd, *adj*. Short of breath
shortwy*n*dyd (1×)

shote, *n*. A muscular spasm of the neck or back; a spasmodic pain in the side, stitch
shote (1×)

shulder, *n*. The shoulder of a person
shuldrys (1×)

shulen, *v*. Shall
shall (13×), shuld (7×), shalt (5×), shulde (4×), shal (3×), shud (1×)

shynen, *v*. To shine
shyny*ng* (5×), shy*n*ny*ng* (4×), shynat (1×)

shynyng, *ng*. The shining of reflected light, brightness
shyny*ng* (1×)

skkyppyng, *ng*. Skipping, jumping, leaping
skkyppyng (1×)

signe, *n*. An indication; proof, evidence
signys (5×), signis (4×), signes (3×), signe (2×), sig*n*is (2×), sign (1×), sygne (1×), syngne (1×)

signifycacion, *n*. A piece of evidence, an indication
signifycac*i*on (1×), signifycacion (1×), signyficacio*u*ns (1×), sygnyficac*i*ons (1×)

signyfien, *v*. To mean, denote
signyfieþ (1×)

sinocha, *n*. A continuous and unintermittent fever
sinocha (1×), sinochus (1×), synoca (1×), synochidem (1×), synocho (1×), Synocus (1×)

siphac, *n*. The peritoneum
Siphac (1×)

skateren, *v*. To scatter; disperse
skateryth (1×)

skye, *n*. A cloud; a nimbus of mist or vapour
skye (8×)

skynne, *n*. The skin
skynne (1×)

skyppyng, *ng*. Skipping, jumping, leaping
skyppyng (1×)

slepe, *n*. A period of sleep
slepe (3×), slepe (1×), sleple (1×)

slepen, *v*. To sleep, be asleep
slepe (1×), slepyng (1×)

slepyng, *ng*. Sleep, the state of being asleep
slepyng (1×)

sloggy, *adj*. Sluggish; characterised by slothfulness
sloggy (1×)

slownesse, *n.* Sluggishness
slownesse (1×)
smale, *adj.* Small
smale (18×), smal (8×), small*er* (1×)
smellen, *v.* To smell
smellyth (2×)
smiten, *v.* To bring about affliction, bring death; cause suffering
smetyn (2×)
smoth, *adj.* Smooth
smoth (2×)
sodenly, *adv.* All at once, suddenly
sodenly (1×)
sodeyn, *adj.* Immediate, prompt, speedy
sodeyn (1×)
sofft, *adj.* Soft
sofft (1×), sofft e (1×)
sofftly, *adv.* Softly
sofftly (2×)
somdel, *adv.* Somewhat, to some degree or extent
somdel (3×)
somwhat, *adv.* Considerably, fully, completely; to some extent or degree; somewhat
somwhat (7×), somwhatt (4×), somewhatt (1×), somwat (1×), somwhatt (1×)
sond, *n.* Sand; a grain of sand
sond (3×)
sondren, *v.* To separate
sondryth (1×)
sonne, *n.* The sun
sonne (2×), soun (2×)
soppe, *n.* A piece of bread dipped or soaked in wine, water, milk, or some other liquid
soppys (1×)
sore, *n.* Pain in bodily parts or organs due to wounds
sor*e* (2×)
sore, *adj.* Painful
sor*e* (1×)
sore, *adv.* Painfully, injuriously
sor*e* (1×)
sorel, *n.* A sour plant, either sour dock or sorrel or wood sorrel
sorel (1×)
sornes, *n.* Physical pain, soreness; suffering
sornes (1×), sornesse (1×)
sorowe, *n.* Physical pain, soreness
sorowe (1×)
sotyl, *adj.* Not dense, light
sotyl (9×), sotyll (1×)
sotylly, *adv.* Delicately, carefully
sotylly (1×)
sotylnesse, *n.* Fineness, thinness, lightness (of a humour) in opposition to thickness, heaviness
sotylnesse (1×)
soule, *n.* Soul
soule (1×)
sounden, *v.* To heal
sownyth (1×)
sourebred, *n.* Leavened bread
sourebred (1×), sowr*e* (1×)
sownyng, *ng.* The ringing or ringing sound in infected ears
sownyng (1×)
sownyth > **sounden**, *v.*
sowre, *adj.* Sour, bitter; phlegm mixed with melancholy, sour phlegm
sowr*e* (1×), sowrysh (1×), sowwer*e* (1×)
soyl, *n.* Soil, the ground in which plants grow
soyl (1×)
space, *n.* Internal space, the area contained within the body or an organ
space (1×)
sparagus, *n.* Asparagus
sp*aragus* (1×)
sparkle, *n.* A small piece of burning material, spark
Sparklis (1×), sp*ar*klys (1×)

spasme, *n.* Violent contraction of muscles, a cramp, spasm
spasme (3×), Spasmus (1×), spasm*us* (1×)
spawd, *n.* The shoulder blade of a person; the human shoulder
spawdys (1×)
Spayn, *n.* The country of Spain
spayn (1×)
special, *adj.* Of special purpose, for some special reason, expressly
special (1×)
specialy, *adv.* Particularly, in particular
specialy (1×)
speken, *v.* To speak
speke (1×)
spermacete, *n.* Ambergris, used medicinally
sp*er*macete (1×)
sperme, *n.* The male seminal fluid
sp*er*me (4×), sp*ar*me (2×), Sparma (1×), sp*ar*ma (1×), Sparma (1×),
spice, *n.* A spice used as a medication or as a medicinal or an alchemical ingredient
spice (17×), spicis (1×), spic*is* (1×)
spirit, *n.* Mental faculties, senses
spi*ri*tis (1×), spirit*is* (1×)
spiritual, *n.* The respiratory organs
sp*iritu*al*is* (4×), sp*iritu*alis (1×), sp*itit*ual (1×)
spiritual, *adj.* Related to the respiratory organs; respiratory
sp*irit*ual (9×), sp*iritu*al (1×), sp*irit*ual (1×), sp*irit*uall (1×), sp*irit*ualys (1×)
spittyng, *ng.* The spitting out of saliva, medicine, etc.
spittyng (1×)
splen, *n.* The spleen of a human
splen (8×), spleen (1×), Splen (1×)
spot, *n.* Any morbid eruption on the skin, a pimple
spott*is* (1×)
spotty, *adj.* Having spots, speckled, mottled in colour, dappled
spotty (1×)
spottyng, *ng.* Spotting of any kind
spottyng (1×)
spuen, *v.* To vomit
spue (1×), spwe (1×)
spume, *n.* Foam, froth
spume (22×), spuma (5×), spwme (3×), spuma (2×)
spumose, *adj.* Full of bubbles, frothy, foamy
spumose (4×)
spumy, *adj.* Foamy
spumy (1×)
spuyng, *ng.* Vomiting
spuyng (1×), spuyng (3×)
spygernel, *n.* Some kind of flowering, broomlike plant used medicinally
spyg*er*nel (1×), Spynegr*e* (1×)
spytten, *v.* To spit
spyttyth (1×)
squame, *n.* The uroscopic content scales, medium-sized flaky particulates suspended in the urine sample
Squame (2×), squames (6×)
stale, *adj.* Not new, clear from having been allowed to settle (beer, wine)
stale (3×)
stampen, *v.* To pound, beat, mash
stampe (2×)
state, *n.* Good physical or emotional condition; good health
state (1×)
stomak, *n.* Stomach
stomak (18×), Stomach*us* (1×), stomak (1×)
ston, *n.* The stone, kidney or bladder stone
ston (14×), stoon (1×)

T

taken, *v.* To take, have
Take (28×), takyn (4×), [T]ake (1×), takyng (1×)

takyng, *ng.* The act of consuming; the act of eating, consuming of food
takyng (2×)

tansy, *n.* The plant tansy
tansy (1×)

taryen, *v.* To delay; to take long to heal
taryet (1×)

tast, *n.* Taste
tast (1×)

techen, *v.* To teach, give training in the methodology or techniques of a science or craft
techyth (1×)

tellen, *v.* To tell, say; inform
tellyllyth (1×)

temperen, *v.* To be mixed, combine, blend
te*m*per*et (1×)

temple, *n.* Temple, the flattened area on either side of the forehead of a human being between the eye and the ear
te*m*plis (1×), templys (1×)

tenasmon, *n.* Tenesmus, a medical condition characterised by a continual urge to defecate, without the ability to do so
tenasmon (4×)

Teophilus, *n.* Theophilus Protospatharius, the seventh-century physician
theo*philus* (10×), theo*philus* (5×), theo*phi*le (2×), theophil*us* (2×), theophile (1×), theophilu*m* (1×), theo*phi*lus (1×), the*ophi*lus (1×), t*heophi*lus (1×), theo*phi*lus (1×), the*ophi*lus (1×)

tercian, *n.* An intermitent fever with paroxysms every third day, counting inclusively (so actually every 48 hours on the first day, then on the third day, then on the fifth day, etc.).
t*er*cian (8×), t*er*cian (1×), t*er*ciana (1×)

terme, *n.* Term, the technical vocabulary associated with a particular field, jargon; a word
terme (2×)

testiculy, *n.* A testicle, testis
testyculy (1×), testiculi (1×), testis (1×)

tete, *n.* A nipple, teat
tetis (1×)

thetanus, *n.* Tetanus, a disease characterised by spasms and rigidity of muscles
Thetan*us* (1×), Thetan*us* (1×)

thicke, *adj.* Thick, dense
thicke (50×), thycke (30×), thick (6×), thyke (4×), thyck (4×), þycke (2×), thicke (1×), thicker (1×), þyck (1×), thycker (1×)

thicknes, *n.* Thickness, denseness
thicknes (1×), thycknesse (1×)

Tholomeus, *n.* The astronomer Ptolemy (c. AD 90–c. 168)
tholome*us* (1×), tholome*us* (1×)

thoutt, *n.* Mental activity; a state of anxiety or distress
thoutt (1×)

throte, *n.* The throat
throte (1×)

throte bolle, *n.* The protuberance of the thyroid cartilage in the front of the human larynx, the Adam's apple
throte bolle (2×)

thrust, *n.* The sensation of thirst, desire to drink
thrust (2×)
thrystyng, *ng.* Pressure, oppression
thrystyng (1×)
thus, *adv.* Thus
thus (1×)
thye, *n.* Thigh
thyes (1×)
thyn, *adj.* Thin, not dense
thy*n*ne (69×), thynne (6×), the*n*ne (2×), thenne (2×), thy*n*ner (2×), thyn (1×), thy*n*ne (1×), thy*n*ne (1×), thy*n*ner*e* (1×)
thyng, *n.* Thing
thyng*is* (3×), thyn (1×), thyng (1×), thyngys (1×)
thynken, *v.* To seem, appear
thynkyth (1×)
thynnen, *v.* To decrease in size, reduce
thy*n*nyth (1×)
thynnhed, *n.* Thinness (of urine)
thy*n*nhed (1×)
to, *n.* A toe of the human foot
toys (1×)
togeder, *adv.* Together
toged*er* (10×), togeder (1×)
token, *n.* Evidence, proof
tokenys (6×), tokyn (6×), token (3×)
tokenyth > **betokenen**, *v.*
torcioun, *n.* A painful twisting of the intestines
torci*ou*n (1×)
tosen, *v.* To tease into a fluffy mass so as to clean and separate the fibers; to separate
tosyd (1×)
touh, *n.* Tow, unworked flax
touh (1×)
towh, *a.* Vioscous, adhesive
towh (1×)
trachearteria, *n.* The tube connecting the larynx and the bronchi, the windpipe; the larynx and trachea taken as a unit
trachearteria (1×)
traueyld, *adj.* Worn out with toil, suffering; exhausted
t*ra*ueyld (1×)
travelen, *v.* To work; give birth; to be afflicted, suffer
t*ra*velyng (2×), t*ra*uel (1×), t*ra*ueyled (1×), t*ra*veylid (1×)
treatise, *n.* Treatise
Treatise (1×)
triacenduli, *n.* An electuary made of three kinds of sandalwood
t*ri*acenduli (1×)
triacle, *n.* An antidote for poison or venom, a medicament for drawing out or neutralising the poison engendered by infection, suppuration, etc.
t*ri*acle (3×), triacle (1×), tryacle (1×)
trobly, *adj.* Dense, turbid, murky
t*ro*bly (15×), trobly (3×)
troblyng, *ng.* Agitation, stirring up; turbulence, storminess
t*ro*bly*n*g (1×)
tuncressed, *n.* The seed of garden cress
tu*n*cressed (1×)
tung, *n.* The tongue
tung (2×)
turmentyl, *n.* The plant tormentil; the root or leaves of this plant used medicinally
t*ur*me*n*tyl (1×), t*ur*mentyl (1×), turmentyll (1×)
turnen, *v.* To change
t*ur*ny*n*g (3×), t*ur*nyth (2×), t*ur*ne (2×), turne (1×), t*ur*nyng (1×)
turnesyke, *n.* Dizziness, faintness, vertigo
t*ur*nesyke (1×)

tyme, *n.* Time
tyme (9×), tyme (1×), tymes (1×)
tympanytes, *n.* A disease in which the abdomen is distended by gas
tympanytes (1×)
tysanne, *n.* A medicinal drink made from shelled barley and water
tysa*nn*ys (1×)
tysyk, *n.* A wasting disease of the lungs, phthisic
tysyk (5×), tesyk (1×), tesyk (3×)

U

vncurabyl, *adj.* Beyond medical help, unable to be cured
vncurabyl (5×)
understonden, *v.* To understand; know
vnd*er*stonde (7×), vnd*er*stond (5×), und*er*stonde (1×)
vngen, *v.* To anoint
vnge (1×)
vnhelthe, *n.* Ill-health, disease
vnhelthe (1×), vnhelþe (1×), onhelthe (1×)
vnkynde, *adj.* Unnatural; uncharacteristic, abnormal
vnkynde (5×), vnky*n*d (1×), onkynde (1×)
vnnethys > **oneþys**, *b.*
vnstabyl, *adj.* Unsteady, shaky, unsure
vnstabyl (1×)
vryn, *n.* Urine
vryn (374×), vryne (2×), vryns (2×), vrina (2×), uryn (1×), uryn (1×), veyn (1×), vrina (3×), vrinys (1×), vrym (1×), vryn (1×), vryn (1×), vry*n* (1×), Urines (1×)
vrynal, *n.* A vessel in which to urinate, a chamber pot
vrynal (5×)
usen, *v.* To use, employ
vse (10×), vsyd (2×)

V

vanden, *v.* To swell, turn, wander, grow dim, become leaden (eyes in leucofleuma)
va*n*dy*n* (1×)
vanyte, *n.* Dizziness, lightheadedness
vanyte (1×), vanyteis (1×)
veneger, *n.* Vinegar, wine vinegar
veneg*er* (1×), vyneg*er* (1×)
ventosyte, *n.* An accumulation of gas in a bodily cavity or organ, flatulence
ventosyte (5×), ventosite (4×), ve*n*tosite (2×)
ventusyng, *ng.* The drawing of blood or other matter by means of a cupping glass, cupping
ventusyng (1×)
ventysshyng, *ng.* Releasing, discharging
ventysshyng (1×)
venymmyng, *ng.* The act of concocting, administering, or applying poison, poison
veny*m*myn*g* (1×)
verdsauce, *n.* A sauce made from green herbs, spices, and wine
v*er*dsauce (1×)
vertu, *n.* Physical strength, power; force, energy
v*er*tu (1×)
verveyne, *n.* A plant of the genus Verbena, vervain
v*er*veyne (1×), v*er*ueyn (1×)

very, *adj.* Reliably indicative, sure
very (1×)

vessel, *n.* A small, portable container
vessel (1×)

vexen, *v.* To afflict physically
vexyd (1×)

veyn, *n.* A vein
veynes (11×), veyne (6×), veyn (1×), veynys (1×)

vice, *n.* An illness, a disorder
vice (4×)

virgyn, *adj.* Fresh, unused, new
v*ir*gyn (1×)

viridis, *adj.* Verdigris, greden like cole juice
viridis (1×), viridis (1×), virid*is* (1×)

viscus quersy, *n.* Mistletoe
visc*us* quersy (1×)

vitrie, *adj.* A congealed and glassy phlegm
vit*rie* (6×), vitres (1×), vitreu*m* (1×), vytrie (1×), vytrye (1×)

vomyte, *n.* An attack or a spell of vomiting
vomyte (1×), vomytys (1×)

voyden, *v.* To purge or relieve of substances
voyde (1×)

vyolet, *n.* A plant of the genus Viola, esp. the sweet violet; the flower of this plant, used medicinally or in cooking
vyolett*is* (1×)

vyscouse, *adj.* Sticky, viscous; dense, thick
vyscouse (8×) viscouse (3×), viscou*s* (1×), visc*us* (1×),

vyscousnesse, *n.* Viscosity
vyscousnesse (1×), viscous-enesse (1×)

W

wakyng, *ng.* Being awake; wakefulness
wakyng (1×)

walle, *n.* A wall (which patients near death tend to pluck at)
walle (1×)

walmyng, *ng.* The churning or roiling of fluids in the body
walmyng (2×), welmyng (1×)

Walterius, *n.* Walter of Agilon, a French physician (c. 1250–1306)
Walt*erius* (19×), Walt*erius* (3×), walt*erium* (1×), walterius (1×), walt*erius* (1×), Walt*erum* (1×), walt*erus* (1×)

walwort, *n.* The plant danewort or dwarf elder; name also applied to other plants: dropwort, chicory or endive, elecampane, hellebore, etc.
walwort (1×)

walwyng, *ng.* Internal upheaval
walwyng (1×), walwyng (1×)

wan, *adj.* Greyish, leaden; dark, black and blue
wan (7×)

wannysh, *adj.* Greyish, whitish grey; leaden; dark
wa*n*nysh (1×), wanysh (1×), wannysh (1×)

war, *adj.* Aware, mindful
war (1×), whar*e* (1×)

warm, *adj.* Warm
warm (1×)

warring, *ng.* Clumpling (together)
warryng (1×)

warysshyng, *ng.* Recovery from illness or injury
warysshyng (10×), waryssyng (4×), warysshsyng (1×)

washen, *v.* To wash, cleanse
wash (1×), wasshyn (1×)

yposarca, *n*. A form of dropsy affecting all of the body, hyposarca
yposarca (1×), yposarcha (1×)

yse, *n*. Ice
yse (1×)

ysodore, *n*. Isidore of Seville (c. 560–636)
ysodore (1×)

ysope, *n*. The herb hyssop
ysope (3×)

ysophagus, *n*. The esophagus
ysophagus (1×)

ytchen, *v*. To feel an itch
ytchyn (1×)

Z

ȝirbus, *n*. A peritoneal serous membrane that envelops the bowels, the greater omentum
ȝirbus (1×)

4. References

Ackerknecht, Erwin H. 1968. *A Short History of Medicine*. Baltimore – London: The Johns Hopkins University Press.

Afnan, Soheil M. 1958. *Avicenna. His Life and Works*. London: George Allen & Unwin.

Alonso-Almeida, Francisco. 2002. "Punctuation Practice in a Late Medieval Medical Remedybook". *Folia Linguistica Historica* 22: 207–232.

Alonso-Almeida, Francisco and Ivalla Ortega-Barrera. 2014. "Sixteenth Century Punctuation in the *Booke of Soueraigne Medicines*". *Onomázein. Revista de lingüística, filología y traducción* 30: 146–168.

Ashtiyani, Saeed Changizi and Ali Cyrus. 2010. "Rhazes, a Genius Physician in Diagnosis and Treatment of Kidney Calculi in Medical History". *Iranian Journal of Kidney Diseases* 4.2: 106–110.

Benskin, Michael. 1991. "The 'Fit'-technique Explained". In Felicity Riddy (ed.). *Regionalism in Late Medieval Manuscripts and Texts: Essays Celebrating the Publication of A Linguistic Atlas of Late Mediaeval English*. Cambridge: D.S. Brewer. 9–26.

Bernstein, William C. 1970. "The Life and Contribution of John Arderne". *Diseases of the Colon and Rectum* 13.1: 8–16.

Blake, Norman. 1996. *A History of the English Language*. Basingstoke – London: Macmillan.

Calle-Martín, Javier. 2004. "Punctuation Practice in a 15th-century Arithmetical Treatise (MS Bodley 790)". *Neuphilologische Mitteilungen* 4: 407–422.

Calle-Martín, Javier. 2011. "Through the Looking Glass: The Palaeography of Benvenutus Grassus' English Vernacular Tradition". In Antonio Miranda-García and Santiago González Fernández-Corugedo (eds.). *Benvenutus Grassus' On the Well-proven Art of the Eye. Practica oculorum & De probatissima arte oculorum. Synoptic Edition and Philological Studies*. Bern: Peter Lang. 35–54.

Calle-Martín, Javier. 2013. "A Middle English Version of *The Doom of Urines* in MS Rawlinson C. 81, ff. 6r–12v". *Analecta Malacitana* 35: 243–274.

Calle-Martín, Javier. 2020. "'*His maiestie chargeth, that no person shall engrose any maner of corne*'. In Merja Kytö and Claudia Claridge (eds.). *Punctuation in Context – Past and Present Perspectives*. Bern: Peter Lang. 179–200.

Calle-Martín, Javier and Antonio Miranda-García. 2005a. "Editing Middle English Punctuation. The Case of MS Egerton 2622 (ff. 136–152)". *International Journal of English Studies* 5.2: 27–44.

Calle-Martin, Javier and Antonio Miranda-García. 2005b. "Aspects of Scribal Punctuation in the Old English Apollonius of Tyre". *Folia Linguistica Historica* 26.1–2: 95–113.

Calle-Martín, Javier and Antonio Miranda-García. 2008. "The Punctuation System of Elizabethan Legal Documents: The Case of G.U.L. MS Hunter 3 (S.1.3)". *The Review of English Studies* 59: 356–378.

Calle-Martín, Javier and Antonio Miranda García. 2012. *The Middle English Version of* De viribus herbarum *(GUL MS Hunter 497, ff. 1r–92r). Edition and Philological Study*. Bern: Peter Lang.

Clemens, Raymond and Timothy Graham. 2007. *Introduction to Manuscript Studies*. Ithaca – London: Cornell University Press.

Cross, Rowin. 2004. *A Handlist of Manuscripts Containing English in the Hunterian Collection Glasgow University Library*. Glasgow: Glasgow University Library.

Cruz-Cabanillas, Isabel de la. 2014. "Punctuation Practice in Manuscript Sainte Geneviève 3390". *Nordic Journal of English Studies* 13.3: 139–159.

Denholm-Young, Noël. 1964. *Handwriting in England and Wales*. Cardiff: University of Wales Press.

Derolez, Albert. 2003. *The Palaeography of Gothic Manuscript Books. From the Twelfth to the Early Sixteenth Century*. Cambridge: Cambridge University Press.

Diepgen, Paul (ed.). 1911. *Gualteri Agilonis Summa medicinalis*. Leipzig: Barth.

Dobson, Eric J. 1957. *English Pronunciation 1500–1700*. 2 vols. Oxford: Clarendon Press.

Eisenberg, Ronald L. 2014. *Essential Figures in Jewish Scholarship*. Lanham: Jason Aronson.

Esteban-Segura, Laura (ed.). 2012. *System of Physic (GUL MS Hunter 509, ff. 1r–167v): A Compendium of Mediaeval Medicine Including the Middle English Gilbertus Anglicus*. Bern: Peter Lang.

Fakhry, Majid. 2001. *Averroes (Ibn Rushd). His Life, Works and Influence*. Oxford: Oneworld Publications.

Fisher, John H. 1996. *The Emergence of Standard English*. Lexington, KY: University Press of Kentucky.

French, Roger. 2003. *Medicine before Science. The Business of Medicine from the Middle Ages to the Enlightenment*. Cambridge: Cambridge University Press.

Getz, Faye Marie. 1990. "Medical Practitioners in Medieval England". *Social History of Medicine* 3.2: 245–283.

Glick, Thomas, Steven J. Livesey and Faith Wallis (eds.). 2005. *Medieval Science, Technology, and Medicine. An Encyclopedia*. New York: Routledge.

Goldberg, Herbert. 2006. *Hippocrates: Father of Medicine*. New York: Authors Choice Press.

González Marrero, José Antonio, María José Martínez Benavides and Paz Fernández Palomeque. 2006. "*De urinis et pulsibus* de Gilles de Corbeil y *De urinis* de Pierleone da Spoleto, un raro de 1514 conservado en la Biblioteca de la Universidad de La Laguna". *Cuadernos de filología clásica* 26.2: 183–192.

Görlach, Manfred. 1991. *Introduction to Early Modern English.* Cambridge: Cambridge University Press.

Hector, Leonard Charles. 1958. *The Handwriting of English Documents.* London: Edward Arnold.

Hope, Jonathan. 2000. "Rats, Bats, Sparrows and Dogs: Biology, Linguistics and the Nature of Standard English". In Laura Wright (ed.). *The Development of Standard English 1300–1800. Theories, Descriptions, Conflicts.* Cambridge: Cambridge University Press. 49–56.

Jacquart, Danielle. 1994. "Medical Practice in Paris in the First Half of the Fourteenth Century". In Luisa García-Ballester, Roger French, Jon Arrizabalaga and Andrew Cunningham (eds.). *Practical Medicine from Salerno to the Black Death.* Cambridge: Cambridge University Press. 186–210.

Jones, Peter Murray. 1989. "Four Middle English Translations of John of Arderne". In Alastair J. Minnis (ed.). *Latin and Vernacular: Studies in Late-Medieval Texts and Manuscripts.* Woodbridge: D.S. Brewer. 61–89.

Jones, Peter Murray. 1994. "John Arderne and the Mediterranean Tradition of Scholastic Surgery". In Luis García-Ballester et al. (eds.). *Practical Medicine from Salerno to the Black Death.* 289–321.

Jones, Peter Murray. 2004. "John Arderne". In H. C. G. Matthew and Brian Harrison (eds.). *Oxford Dictionary of National Biography.* Oxford: Oxford University Press. http://www.oxforddnb.com/view/article/636?docPos=1 (accessed March 2, 2015).

Ker, Neil R. 1983. *Medieval Manuscripts in British Libraries, vol. III, Lampeter-Oxford.* Oxford: Clarendon Press.

Kors, Alan Charles and Edward Peters. 2001. *Witchcraft in Europe, 400–1700. A Documentary History.* Philadelphia: University of Pennsylvania Press.

Kouba, Eric, Eric M. Wallen and Sridhar Raj Pruthi. 2007. "Uroscopy by Hippocrates and Theophilus: Prognosis versus Diagnosis". *Journal of Urology* 177.1: 50.52

Kurath, Hans, Hereman M. Kuhn and Robert. E. Lewis. 2001. *The Electronic Version of the Middle English Dictionary.* Ann Arbor, Michigan: University of Michigan Press.

Latham, Ronald E., David R. Howlett and Richard K. Ashdowne. 1975–. *Dictionary of Medieval Latin from British Sources.* Oxford: British Academy. Accessible via the Longeion website <http://logeion.uchicago.edu/index.html>.

Lester, Godfrey Allen. 1985. *The Index of Middle English Prose. Handlist 2, a Handlist of Manuscripts Containing Middle English Prose in the John Rylands University Library of Manchester and Chetham's Library, Manchester.* Cambridge: Brewer.

Taavitsainen, Irma and Päivi Pahta. 2004. "Vernacularisation of Scientific and Medical Writing in Its Sociohistorical Context". In Irma Taavitsainen and Päivi Pahta (eds.). *Medical and Scientific Writing in Late Medieval English.* Cambridge: Cambridge University Press. 1–22.

Tannenbaum, Samuel A. 1930. *The Handwriting of the Renaissance.* New York: University Press.

Tavormina, M. Teresa. 2005. "The Twenty-Jordan Series: An Illustrated Middle English Uroscopy Text". *ANQ: A Quarterly Journal of Short Articles, Notes and Reviews* 18.3: 43–67.

Tavormina, M. Teresa. 2007a. "A Newly-Identified Copy of John Arderon's De Judiciis Urinarum". Paper presented at the *Annual Meeting of the Early Book Society.* Salford, UK.

Tavormina, M. Teresa. 2007b. "The Middle English *Letter of Ipocras*". *English Studies* 88.6: 632–652.

Tavormina, M. Teresa. 2010. "Three Middle English Verse Uroscopies". *English Studies* 91.6: 591–622.

Tavormina, M. Teresa. 2014. "Uroscopy in Middle English. A Guide to the Texts and Manuscripts". *Studies in Medieval and Renaissance History* 3.11: 1–154.

Tronch-Perez, Jesús (ed.). 2002. *A Synoptic Hamlet: A Critical-Synoptic Edition of the Second Quarto and First Folio Texts of* Hamlet. Valencia: Universidad de Valencia.

Trudgill, Peter. 1999. "Standard English: what it isn't". In Tony Bex and Richard J. Watts (eds.). *Standard English: the Widening Debate.* London – New York: Routledge. 117–128.

Vieillard, Camille. 1903. *L'urologie et les médecins urologues dans la médecine ancienne: Gilles de Corbeil: sa vie, ses oeuvres, son poème des urines.* Paris: F. de Rudeval.

Wallis, Faith. 2005. "Gilles of Corbeil". In Thomas Glick, Steven J. Livesey and Faith Wallis (eds.). *Medieval Science, Technology and Medicine: an Encyclopedia.* New York: Routledge. 198.

Wickersheimer, Ernest. 1979. *Dictionnaire biographique des médicins en France au Moyen Âge.* Genève: Librairie Droz.

Young, John and P. Henderson Aitken. 1908. *A Catalogue of the Manuscripts in the Library of the Hunterian Museum in the University of Glasgow.* Glasgow: James Maclehose and Sons.

Zimmerman, Leo M. and Ilza Veith. 1993. *Great Ideas in the History of Surgery.* San Francisco: Norman Publishing.

Printed and bound by CPI Group (UK) Ltd, Croydon, CR0 4YY

13/09/2026

14960648-0002